The Complete Guide to
Food Allergies
in Adults and Children

A Johns Hopkins Press Health Book

The 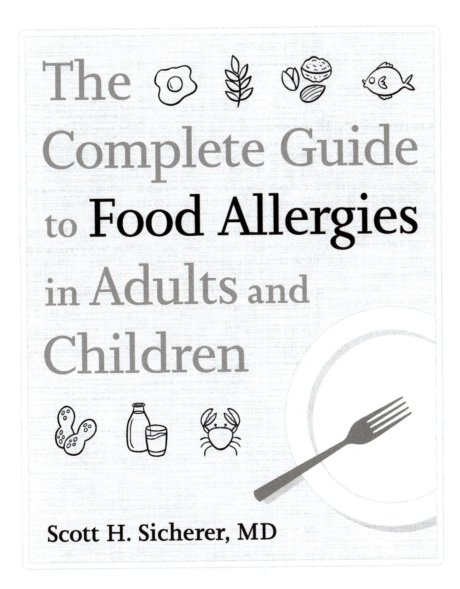 Complete Guide to **Food Allergies** in Adults and Children

Scott H. Sicherer, MD

JOHNS HOPKINS UNIVERSITY PRESS

Baltimore

Note to the Reader: This book is not meant to substitute for medical care, and treatment should not be based solely on its contents. Instead, treatment must be developed in a dialogue between the individual and their physician. Our book has been written to help with that dialogue.

Drug dosage: The author and publisher have made reasonable efforts to determine that the selection of drugs discussed in this text conform to the practices of the general medical community. The medications described do not necessarily have specific approval by the US Food and Drug Administration for use in the diseases for which they are recommended. In view of ongoing research, changes in governmental regulation, and the constant flow of information relating to drug therapy and drug reactions, the reader is urged to check the package insert of each drug for any change in indications and dosage and for warnings and precautions. This is particularly important when the recommended agent is a new and/or infrequently used drug.

Johns Hopkins University Press
2715 North Charles Street
Baltimore, Maryland 21218-4363
www.press.jhu.edu

Library of Congress Cataloging-in-Publication Data

Names: Sicherer, Scott H., author.
Title: The complete guide to food allergies in adults and children /
   Scott H. Sicherer, MD.
Description: Baltimore : Johns Hopkins University Press, 2022. |
   Series: A Johns Hopkins press health book | Includes index.
Identifiers: LCCN 2021017979 | ISBN 9781421443140 (hardcover) |
   ISBN 9781421443157 (paperback) | ISBN 9781421443164 (ebook)
Subjects: LCSH: Food allergy. | Food allergy in children. | Food allergy—
   Treatment. | Food allergy—Prevention. | Self-care, Health.
Classification: LCC RC596 .S378 2022 | DDC 616.97/5—dc23
LC record available at https://lccn.loc.gov/2021017979

A catalog record for this book is available from the British Library.

Special discounts are available for bulk purchases of this book. For more information, please contact Special Sales at specialsales@jh.edu.

Contents

CHAPTER 6
Mastering Allergen Avoidance   159

CHAPTER 7
Maintaining Lifestyle and Quality of Life, Reducing Anxiety, and Keeping a Healthy Diet   204

CHAPTER 8
The Natural Course and Resolution of Food Allergies   222

Preface

This book is dedicated to people with food allergies and those who care for them. It is the result of thousands of questions I have been asked by adults and children with food allergies; parents of children with food allergies; as well as allergists, medical students, physicians in training, pediatricians, the media, government officials, researchers, teachers, school nurses, and others. Your questions have led me at times to seek answers from you as well as from others, from research, and through trial and error. It is my pleasure and privilege to present this book, which is designed to give you what you have asked for: a place to find accurate, timely, detailed, and helpful answers to questions on every aspect of food allergies.

I marvel at the amazing strides I have witnessed in the diagnosis, prevention, and treatment of food allergies, particularly over the past five years. We now have tests that are better at diagnosing a true allergy, and even better ones are on the way. We have gained insights on how food allergy can be prevented, with a clear approach for peanut, and are in the midst of multiple studies on preventing other food allergies. The first therapy for food allergy approved by the US Food and Drug Administration, a peanut oral immunotherapy product, has come into practice. In parallel, oral immunotherapy approaches to other foods are under study and are also being used in many practices. Numerous exciting novel approaches are also under study, with increasingly better safety and efficacy. In this book, I explore all of these areas to help you make informed decisions. While the emerging therapies are presenting some difficult choices, they also offer a remarkable number of options to treat food allergy and improve quality of life. It is hard for me to imagine, based on what I see in this field, that we will be doing what we are doing now in another five or ten years. I feel confident in telling my young patients that when they are adults, they may not need to avoid the foods they are allergic to today. Although most of the approaches that are emerging are not a simple "cure," I have strong hope that we will get there.

This book would not exist were it not for the work and influences of many people, and so I dedicate this book to the many who have taught me over the years, including Hugh A. Sampson, MD; Sally Noone, RN; Marion

Groetch, RD; and Robert A. Wood, MD. It is also dedicated to my many colleagues at Mount Sinai's Jaffe Food Allergy Institute, and researchers and colleagues worldwide. I want to thank the National Institute of Allergy and Infectious Diseases and Food Allergy Research & Education for supporting my research. I thank the Jaffe family for their foresight in establishing a food allergy institute at Mount Sinai in New York, and also the many families and visionary philanthropists for supporting our research and clinical care initiatives. Most importantly, I thank the children, adults, and families who have altruistically contributed to our understanding of food allergy by their participation in research studies—they are absolutely the heroes who will help us to cure this disease. Finally, I thank my wife, Mati, and children, Andrew, Zachary, Maya, Sydnee, and Cassaddee . . . for everything.

Introduction

Hugh A. Sampson, MD
Emeritus Director, Jaffe Food Allergy Institute,
Icahn School of Medicine at Mount Sinai, New York

Over the past four decades, I have been fortunate to witness and participate in a remarkable evolution in our understanding of food allergies. When I began my food allergy research in the early 1980s, I approached the disorder by applying my background in detailed scientific methods. Although a bit reluctant and highly skeptical, I was encouraged to explore this area by Dr. Susan Dees, an emeritus professor and a wonderful mentor during my early years at Duke University. Then my own fascination with the field grew as a result of experiences with my second daughter, who had food allergies, eczema, and later asthma, and as I cared for an increasing number of families and children with food allergy symptoms in my clinical practice. In those early years, I was reluctant to admit to my colleagues that I was focusing my research on food allergy. The reason for my trepidation was that food allergy, in those early days, was considered not a "real disease" but a problem of little consequence. Part of the reason for this misperception was that many people were attributing various problems to foods that were never proven to be involved using scientifically validated methods. At the same time, people were not recognizing allergic diseases that actually were caused or worsened by foods. Although everyone acknowledged that a food could cause a severe allergic reaction, the life-threatening nature of this allergy was not well appreciated.

In the mid-1970s, the food allergy field began to emerge from scientific uncertainty in part because of the work of Drs. Charles May and Allan Bock, who emphasized the need to use a diagnostic procedure called a *double-blind, placebo-controlled oral food challenge*, which is discussed in detail in this book. This test brought objectivity to the diagnosis of food allergies by eliminating patients' and physicians' preconceived notions. In my research work, the procedure fostered incredible scientific advances to further improve the diagnosis and treatment of food allergies. Food allergy became "real" and was now viewed as a medical illness worthy of attention and acknowledged as a field of allergy in need of more research. Today, food allergy has become a hot topic, and many programs around the world are actively pursuing a better understanding of these disorders and effective forms of prevention and therapy. This expanded involvement by the scientific community has resulted in the topic of food allergy dominating sessions and abstract presentations at international congresses held throughout the world.

The emergence of food allergy from the "dark ages" into a time of scientific exploration was exciting; however, the past decades have unfortunately witnessed an alarming increase in food allergies and other allergic diseases. All ages are affected. The burden of living with food allergies remains largely untold and underappreciated. Those who are allergic and their families must practice constant dietary caution and be at the ready to treat severe allergic reactions. Despite increasing awareness, this disease is still sometimes fatal.

The good news is that the past decade has witnessed a revolution in the approach to food allergy. Diagnostics have improved to reduce the need for oral food challenges. Proven approaches to preventing food allergy are in practice with more to come. Multiple therapies are under study and in use, including a first FDA-approved treatment. Amazing basic science advances are leading the way to new and better modalities to predict, prevent, and treat food allergy. The dizzying array of options and new approaches can be confusing.

The explosion of information (and misinformation) about food allergy has outpaced our ability to teach food allergy sufferers, parents, children, and caregivers what we have learned and what they need to know. Being unable to find reliable information with sufficient details about food allergies leaves patients and their families feeling unfulfilled and confused. They have many burning questions and concerns. We now have clear answers for many of these concerns, and when the right answer is unclear, we have plenty of information that can be helpful while research is underway. Knowing the answers and understanding the issues behind what we can and cannot yet answer are vital to working with your doctor, discussing your or your child's food allergy with others, and ultimately obtaining the best care possible. This book is an encyclopedia of the essential information you need to do this, and it is the only resource I know of that provides timely, accurate, and accessible information on every medical aspect of food allergy.

Dr. Scott Sicherer, an internationally recognized leader in food allergy education and research, has culled nearly three decades of experience in patient care and research to present this information in a readable and understandable format. He provides both basic medical information and tips on how to deal with everyday issues such as visiting the allergist; going to school, work, and restaurants; and navigating the supermarket. Dr. Sicherer has been at the cutting edge of clinical and social issues of food allergy. As a lecturer, he has had countless discussions about food allergy experiences with patients, parents, school nurses, camp directors, food service professionals, pediatricians, internists, allergists, children, and many others. He has distilled these experiences here to answer virtually every possible question about food allergies, from questions you may have wondered about to, even more importantly, many questions you should be asking.

The information in this book is so comprehensive and timely that it should be required reading not only for adults with food allergies and parents of children with food allergies, but also for physicians, teachers, school nurses, camp personnel, spouses, and everyone who plays a role in caring for those with food allergies. It will help them to understand and more effectively and safely manage these allergies, and to understand emerging treatment and prevention strategies. I certainly plan to keep a copy in my clinic and to recommend it to the many people I encounter whose lives are affected in some way by pervasive allergies to food.

The Complete Guide to
Food Allergies
in Adults and Children

CHAPTER 1

Understanding Food Allergy and Intolerance

Food is our sustenance, but it can also make us sick in a variety of ways. This chapter describes food allergy (a focus of this book), food intolerance, and other ways that food can cause problems.

Food Allergy

What is a food allergy?

A food allergy happens when the immune system, a part of the body that usually fights germs, attacks harmless proteins in foods.

How does the immune system "attack" proteins in foods?

Two ways: with cells that release various chemicals, and by producing proteins called IgE antibodies.

What role do the IgE antibodies play in food allergy?

The most common forms of food allergy, when allergic reactions happen suddenly after a food is eaten, are the result of the immune system making IgE antibodies. These proteins are like small antennae that sit atop allergy cells (called mast cells and basophils) and detect the food proteins. The IgE "antennae" are able to detect a specific food protein, for example, a peanut protein or an egg protein. When these IgE antibodies come in contact with the food protein, they signal the allergy cells to release powerful chemicals, such as histamine, which produce allergic symptoms.

How do cells in the immune system cause food allergies?

The cells respond to the food protein by releasing chemicals that cause inflammation with persistent symptoms, such as rashes, or symptoms affecting the gut, such as pain, nausea, and vomiting. The term "non-IgE-mediated," or "cell-mediated," food allergy is used when the cells of the immune system are causing allergic responses to foods without involving IgE.

Other than food allergy, how might foods make a person sick?

A food can make a person ill in many ways. Food poisoning happens when bacteria in spoiled food release toxins that can cause symptoms. Chemicals in foods can cause symptoms in some people. For example, caffeine may cause sweating, tremors, or heart palpitations. Food intolerance causes some people to become ill from a food that does not trouble others.

At what age does a person develop a food allergy?

Any age. Food allergies most often develop in infancy and childhood, however.

What are the most common triggers of food allergy in infants, children, and adults?

For infants and children, cow's milk, eggs, and peanuts are the most common triggers, followed by tree nuts, shellfish, soy, wheat, and fish. Adult-onset food allergy usually involves nuts, seafood, fruits, or vegetables.

How do I know if I have a food allergy?

Specific symptoms after eating a food, or patterns of symptoms, are a good clue that you may have a food allergy. These will be described below.

Food Intolerance, Irritable Bowel Syndrome, and Celiac Disease

What is a food intolerance?

Strictly speaking, "food intolerance" typically refers to trouble digesting specific food ingredients because of deficiency in enzymes, resulting in symptoms affecting the gut. But the terms "intolerance" and "sensitivity" are often used to describe a host of problems experienced from foods that are distinct from food allergy. In a broader sense, food intolerances or sensitivities are terms often used to include not only problems with digestion (the best example being lactose intolerance), but also irritable bowel syndrome, problems caused by food additives, celiac disease, and even stress-related problems associated with foods. While not usually falling under the definition of "intolerance," a person with gall bladder disease may notice problems with fatty foods and consider themselves to be "sensitive" to them. A person with gout may consider themselves sensitive to certain meats and seafood, as they can contribute to the disease. Here we discuss classical food intolerance and irritable bowel syndrome (IBS) and celiac disease. Later in this chapter we review problems attributed to chemical properties of foods and food additives.

What are differences between food allergy and intolerance?

Aside from the distinction that allergy involves the immune system and intolerance does not (an exception is celiac disease, which is sometimes called gluten-sensitive enteropathy), the symptoms differ in some ways but can overlap. Typical symptoms of intolerance affect the gut (pain, vomit, diarrhea). While food allergy symptoms may also involve the gut, they can include life-threatening symptoms that affect breathing and blood circulation as well. Another distinction is that many people with intolerance can get by eating small or modest amounts of problem foods, while many people with food allergies react to small amounts.

What is lactose intolerance?

A difficulty in digesting the sugar, called lactose, in milk, because of a deficiency in an enzyme called lactase, is called lactose intolerance. Without sufficient lactase enzyme, the lactose passes along the intestine undigested and unabsorbed. Gut bacteria can take hold of the lactose and ferment it, causing gas. The extra sugar in the intestine can draw fluids out of the body and into the gut, causing diarrhea.

Who is at risk for lactose intolerance?

After infancy and early childhood, most of us gradually lose our ability to digest lactose. Having a lactase deficiency in adulthood is actually a normal situation, although the degree varies among different races and ethnicities. Persons of Asian descent have the highest rates of lactase deficiency, over 90%. Of Native Americans and African Americans, more than 70% have lactase deficiency. The lowest rates, 5% to 20%, are among white adults. The rate at which lactase levels decrease over time as a person ages is also racially and ethnically related. For example, within a few years after breast-feeding, Chinese and Japanese lose 80% to 90% of lactase, while Jews and Asians lose 60% to 70%. White northern Europeans may reach their lowest level of lactase after age 20. Having a stomach virus can also result in temporary loss of lactase for days or weeks.

What foods cause symptoms of lactose intolerance?

Any food with milk. Dairy products normally contain about 4% to 5% lactose by weight, enough to create symptoms in lactose intolerant people. However, different foods may have different amounts. Cheese and yogurt often do not lead to symptoms because lactic acid bacteria in the foods help to digest the lactose. Some cheeses contain less lactose, including camembert, cheddar, cream cheese, and parmesan.

How much milk sugar causes symptoms when a person has lactose intolerance?

This is quite variable, with some people being sensitive to tiny amounts and others being able to have many ounces before symptoms appear.

How is lactose intolerance diagnosed?

Usually through trial and error, by seeing if reducing lactose in the diet relieves symptoms. But a medical diagnosis can be confirmed with testing, using a breath hydrogen test performed by drinking lactose and having a breath test to check for poor absorption.

How is lactose intolerance treated?

By reducing the lactose. This is accomplished either by dietary reduction or avoidance, purchasing lactose-free milk products, or using replacement enzymes that are available over the counter. It is helpful to be familiar with dairy products that have high or low lactose content (see table 1.1).

What other foods cause this type of intolerance?

Beans contain a sugar that is hard to digest, giving them a reputation for causing gas. That is why supplements containing enzymes are sold to reduce gas from eating beans. Some people have trouble absorbing a sugar called fructose, especially in foods with lower amounts of glucose, another

Table 1.1. Lactose Content of Dairy Foods

Dairy Foods with High Lactose Content	Dairy Foods with Low Lactose Content
Whole milk (condensed, evaporated, liquid)	Hard cheeses (cheddar, parmesan, Swiss)
Ice cream	Butter
Cottage cheese	Sour cream
Buttermilk	Cream cheese
Goat's milk	Lactose-free milk and yogurts
Conventional yogurt	Kefir
	Some yogurts (probiotic, Greek)
	Heavy cream

sugar. The symptoms can include gas, diarrhea, and abdominal pain. Problem foods include apples, artichokes, fruit juices, high-fructose corn syrup, honey, leeks, onions, pears, raisins, sorbitol, watermelon, and wheat. A doctor can diagnose this problem using a breath hydrogen test.

Can a person be intolerant of alcohol?

Some people (particularly Asians) are unable to properly digest alcohol. The by-products cause symptoms that can include skin redness, nausea, vomiting, sleepiness, and sometimes a wheeze. The same effect sometimes happens when alcohol and certain medications are being used at the same time. Some medications that affect how the body processes alcohol are the antibiotic metronidazole (Flagyl) and the antifungal medication griseofulvin (Fulvicin or Grifulvin). Drinking alcohol while using a skin cream called Elidel or Protopic causes a peculiar reaction in some people, who develop skin redness where they applied the cream.

Can food intolerance be dangerous?

Usually not. There are some specific hereditary illnesses where metabolism or digestion of dietary components can cause extreme symptoms, however. An example is hereditary fructose intolerance, where seizures and liver

damage can occur. Another example is glucose-6-phosphate dehydroge-
nase deficiency, where anemia and blood problems can occur from fava
beans, red wine, and certain medications.

What is irritable bowel syndrome?

Irritable bowel syndrome, also known as IBS, is diagnosed when there is
a failure to identify medical illnesses contributing to a constellation of
symptoms that include stomach pain, discomfort, and either constipation
or diarrhea. About one in eight people have these symptoms. Different
subtypes are identified. Some include mostly diarrhea, others constipation,
and others alternating constipation and diarrhea. Sometimes the illness develops after an infection. IBS tends to be chronic and affects quality of life.

What causes irritable bowel syndrome?

There are many theories about the causes, from infections to stress. Your
doctor should consider medical illnesses that could cause the symptoms, including infection, celiac disease, and inflammatory bowel diseases. Treatments
include medications, psychotherapy, probiotics, and dietary alterations.

Is irritable bowel syndrome caused by food allergies?

Food allergy is one problem to consider when an individual experiences
some of the symptoms of IBS. A recent study suggested that for some
people with IBS, foods are causing an isolated allergic reaction in the gut,
but studies have not identified food allergy as a primary cause of the syndrome itself. A person with symptoms of IBS should be thoroughly evaluated to exclude many illnesses that can cause the symptoms. The terms food
"sensitivity" or "intolerance" are sometimes used because dietary alterations
can improve IBS symptoms despite absence of true allergy.

What role does food play in irritable bowel syndrome?

A number of studies have tried to use various elimination diets, some with
success, although careful studies are lacking. A traditional approach to diet
in persons with IBS suggests avoiding large meals, having a regular daily
pattern of meals, and reducing intake of fat, insoluble fibers, caffeine, and
gassy foods. Contributing problems of lactose intolerance or other sugar
intolerances may be responsible and should be considered. Reducing or
eliminating milk or wheat may result in a diet that favors the consumption
of foods that promote better digestion, such as fruits and vegetables. A low

Table 1.2. Inflammatory Bowel Syndrome and the FODMAPS Diet

What to Consider When Using a Low FODMAPS Diet for IBS	Restricted Foods	Foods That Are Not Restricted
Verify your diagnosis Talk to your doctor about treatments Consider simpler diets ahead of FODMAPS Keep a food diary, and consider re-expanding the diet gradually, because not all foods may be problematic or may be tolerated in moderation Work with a registered dietitian	Apple, asparagus, beans, cashew, cauliflower, cherry, garlic, high-fructose corn syrup, leek, milk, mushroom, onion, pear, pistachio, raisin, watermelon, wheat/gluten	Almond, beef, brown rice, carrot, chicken, coconut oil, egg, fenugreek, fish, grape, lactose-free milk products, mustard, oat, olive, olive oil, orange, pepper, potato, quinoa, strawberry, tofu, walnut

FODMAPS diet may also be trialed. FODMAPS stands for **F**ermentable **O**ligosaccharides, **D**isaccharides, **M**onosaccharides **A**nd **P**olyols. Table 1.2 shows foods that are restricted on a FODMAPS diet and provides information about pursuing the diet. It appears that supplementation with soluble fiber, such as psyllium, can improve IBS symptoms for many sufferers. Insoluble fiber such as cellulose may be unhelpful. Discuss any diet or medication with your health care professional.

Can IgG tests identify foods causing IBS?

As discussed in chapter 3, the IgG or IgG4 protein represents a normal immune response to foods. Studies have not convincingly shown that such testing can identify food triggers in IBS. Although dietary alterations may be one means to address IBS (along with fiber, medications, stress reduction, and so on), these specific tests are not proven.

What is celiac disease?

Celiac disease is caused by an immune system response to gluten, a protein in wheat, and related proteins in barley and rye. The disorder is also called gluten-sensitive enteropathy. This is an inherited disorder affecting the gut and sometimes other parts of the body. Nearly 1 in 100 persons has celiac disease.

Is celiac disease a food allergy?

Although celiac disease is caused by an abnormal immune response to gluten, most experts do not consider this to be a typical food allergy because the symptoms are so different.

How does celiac disease differ from a wheat allergy?

Wheat allergy results in rapid, typical symptoms of allergy, such as hives and swelling. Unfortunately, unlike most food allergies, celiac disease symptoms are chronic, and the disease does not resolve. Celiac disease is also associated with a risk for cancer.

When is celiac disease suspected?

The diagnosis of celiac disease is considered if there are symptoms such as diarrhea, poor growth, stomach pain, vomiting, constipation, bloating, and irritability. Since this disease is inherited, suspicion is higher if other family members have celiac disease. Sometimes there are symptoms outside of the gut, for example, poorly developed tooth enamel, blistering skin rashes, and poor bone development.

How is celiac disease diagnosed?

Blood tests can be done if a person is currently eating gluten-containing grains. Genetic testing may also help determine a diagnosis. The most accurate method of diagnosis requires a biopsy of the gut.

How is celiac disease treated?

By strict avoidance of gluten.

What is "non-celiac gluten sensitivity"?

This term has been used to describe people without medical evidence of celiac disease who experience some symptoms of celiac disease and have a response to gluten avoidance. Some experts suspect that this condition may be caused by a different type of intolerance related to sugars, and not directly to gluten, or may be a form of irritable bowel disease or mild wheat allergy. A thorough evaluation by a gastroenterologist is recommended to ensure a correct diagnosis.

Food Allergy Symptoms and Illnesses

What symptoms should make me suspect a food allergy?

Having sudden allergic symptoms within an hour or two of eating a food should raise suspicions of a food allergy. But allergic reactions can also be more insidious. A food allergy can cause chronic daily symptoms that may be more difficult to connect to particular foods.

What are common sudden symptoms of a food allergy?

Sudden allergic symptoms (also called acute symptoms) can affect the skin with rashes such as hives (like mosquito bites), swelling (especially of the face and lips), itching, and flaring of eczema rashes. Symptoms can affect breathing with throat tightness, repetitive coughing, wheezing, swelling of the throat and tongue, difficulty swallowing, and trouble getting air in and out. The gut can be affected with pain, nausea, vomiting, and diarrhea. There may be itchiness in the mouth and throat, or an odd taste such as a metallic one. Women may feel uterine contractions. When blood circulation is impaired, the heart may beat very fast or very slow, the skin may turn pale or blue, the pulse may be difficult to feel, blood pressure may be low, and there can be confusion, dizziness, light-headedness, and passing out. Sometimes in a severe allergic reaction, a person has a feeling of impending doom.

What are common chronic symptoms of a food allergy?

When foods cause a constant inflammation in the body, the person may have chronic rashes of allergic eczema, also called atopic dermatitis. There may be gut symptoms of vomiting, pain, or diarrhea; poor growth in children; or weight loss in adults.

What types of medical illnesses are caused by food allergy?

Several medical illnesses result from sudden or chronic food-allergic reactions. These go by many different medical terms, including anaphylaxis, oral allergy syndrome, eczema, proctocolitis, enterocolitis, enteropathy, eosinophilic esophagitis, contact hives, occupational food allergy, food-associated exercise-induced anaphylaxis (FAEIA), and others. I devote entire chapters in this book to considering the details of many of these problems.

What is anaphylaxis?

Anaphylaxis is a severe allergic reaction that is rapid in onset and can be fatal. Typically, several areas of the body are affected, for example, the skin and the gut, or the gut and breathing. Chapter 4 is devoted to questions about anaphylaxis.

What is oral allergy syndrome / pollen-associated food allergy syndrome?

A person with this type of allergy is initially allergic to proteins in pollens and then has symptoms when eating certain raw fruits or vegetables that have similar proteins in them (not on them). A pollen-allergic person would not normally clean a pollen-covered car by licking it, but if he did, his tongue might get very itchy. Biting into an apple that is rich with pollen-like proteins can lead to the same uncomfortable mouth symptoms. The problem occurs only with raw forms of fruits and vegetables because heating the food destroys the problematic proteins.

What are examples of the pollen and food relationships?

Table 1.3 provides some of the relationships of pollens and foods. Most of the allergic relationships are mild and only involve the raw forms of the foods. Importantly, it is possible to have allergy to many of the listed foods without the allergy being related to pollens (for example, peanut allergy), and some allergies can be severe. While ragweed pollen proteins are related to melons and bananas and grass pollens are related to some grains like wheat, whether there is illness caused by these relationships is controversial. Many people with pollen allergies have no symptoms, and those who do have symptoms vary greatly from each other in which foods bother them.

Can oral allergy syndrome be severe?

Rarely. About 1% or 2% experience more severe reactions, and about 7% have symptoms beyond the mouth. One reason reactions are usually mild is that people generally stop eating the food if it bothers them too much.

Can a person with oral allergy syndrome eat the food anyway?

Many people with oral allergy syndrome eat the raw foods if they are not too uncomfortable. Additionally, the heated forms of these foods (applesauce, canned fruits, cooked carrots, peach pie, etc.) should be tolerated.

Table 1.3. Relationships of Pollen to Foods

Pollen	Foods That May Be Involved
Birch	Almond, apple, carrot, celery, cherry, hazel, jackfruit, kiwi, mung bean, peach, peanut, pear, Sharon fruit, soy, strawberry
Olive tree	Kiwi, latex, melon, olive, peach, pear
Plane tree	Apple, chickpea, corn, hazel, kiwi, lettuce, peach, peanut
Cypress tree	Peach
Ficus tree	Avocado, banana, fig, kiwi, latex, papaya, pineapple
Mugwort	Aniseed, cabbage, caraway seed, carrot, cauliflower, celery, coriander seed, corn, fennel seed, garlic, grape, leek, mango, mustard, onion, paprika, parsley, pepper, sunflower

How can food be rendered less likely to trigger a reaction in oral allergy syndrome?

The easiest means is to heat the food. Some people get relief from symptoms by briefly microwaving, peeling, or dipping the food in lemon juice.

Is there seasonal variation in oral allergy syndrome?

The symptoms tend to increase during the relevant pollen season and fade or improve after. Therefore, when your eyes and nose are itchiest in the pollen season, you are more apt to have problems eating the related raw fruits or vegetables. When you are at the longest period away from your pollen season—just before the season begins the following year—the symptoms from eating the problem foods should be at their minimum.

Why do some foods bother a person with oral allergy syndrome and other related ones do not?

It is remarkable that people with the same pollen allergy can have symptoms with different related foods or with none at all. We do not know the reason for this variation.

Can a person with oral allergy symptoms from one type of apple tolerate different types?

Surprisingly, yes. For example, a person may have no symptoms from Fuji apples but become quite itchy from Granny Smith apples. This is probably because different types of apples vary in the amounts of the relevant proteins as well as in the degree of similarity to the pollens. Additionally, the allergenic proteins tend to increase with longer storage times, so fresher apples may be less of a problem.

How do doctors treat oral allergy syndrome?

Allergists differ in whether they have their patients avoid these foods, with many making case-by-case decisions based on the person's history of reactions. For example, the more discomfort someone has felt, the more likely a doctor will advise the person to avoid the food. Taking antihistamines might reduce symptoms. Some studies suggest that immunotherapy (allergy shots) against the related pollens may also reduce symptoms.

Are symptoms of oral allergy to nuts more concerning?

Nuts are in general more likely than fruits and vegetables to cause severe allergic reactions. Some nuts have pollen-related proteins and fall into the same category as other pollen-related food allergens, however, perhaps indicating less risk of a severe reaction. Almonds, hazelnuts, and peanuts have pollen-related proteins, so they may cause relatively mild allergies for some people. Since these foods are known to trigger severe reactions, however, an allergist may suggest that a person who's had any symptoms should avoid them entirely.

What is food-related atopic dermatitis, or eczema?

Atopic dermatitis, or allergic eczema, is a chronic skin condition in which the skin is dry, rashy, and very itchy. About one in three children with worse-than-mild forms of the rash also have food allergies.

What are proctocolitis, enterocolitis, and enteropathy?

These are gut allergies that usually begin in infancy and have symptoms such as vomiting, diarrhea (sometimes bloody), pain, and poor growth, depending on the particular illness. Most people outgrow these types of allergies during childhood. Cow's milk is the most common trigger.

What are eosinophilic esophagitis and eosinophilic gut disease?

Eosinophilic gut disease results from a chronic allergic inflammation in the lining of the digestive tract. Swelling and breakdown of the gut lining result in symptoms, which vary depending on what area of the gut has swelling. For example, inflammation in the esophagus (eosinophilic esophagitis), the tube connecting the mouth to the stomach, causes pain when food is swallowed, and food may get stuck in the tube. For most people with this illness, food is the main trigger of the inflammation.

What are contact hives?

When a food touches the skin directly and results in hives where the food made contact, these are called contact hives, also known as contact urticaria. This term is usually reserved for situations when a food, although tolerated when eaten, causes symptoms only on skin contact. Contact urticaria occurs most often in infants and young children, when messy eating results in hives around the mouth but the food is otherwise tolerated. Common triggers are acidic fruits, such as tomatoes and strawberries.

What is food-associated exercise-induced anaphylaxis?

People with this problem can exercise without any allergic symptoms. They can also eat without symptoms. But if they eat foods, or a particular food, and then exercise, they develop allergic symptoms and possibly anaphylaxis. Common triggers are celery, shellfish, and wheat.

What are occupational food allergies?

These allergies are related to exposure on the job, usually to large amounts of food, and often through the skin or air. Baker's asthma describes a situation where wheat flour in the air triggers wheezing, although the baker can eat wheat products. People working with fruits or vegetables might develop skin rashes from the exposure, with the rashes flaring from skin contact with the food. Many different foods can cause occupation-related reactions.

Severity

How severe can a food allergy be?

Food allergies can be fatal.

Do allergic reactions worsen each time a food is eaten?

No. This is a common misconception. Subsequent reactions could be more severe, less severe, or equal in severity.

Is severity of a food allergy predictable?

No, although there are some patterns. Certain foods are more likely to cause dangerous reactions. For example, peanut, tree nut, shellfish, and fish allergies are usually more severe than fruit or vegetable allergies. Severity may be related to the amount eaten, with more dangerous symptoms following a larger amount ingested. Having coexisting asthma is also a risk factor for more extreme reactions.

Why is having asthma a risk factor for more severe reactions?

Asthma is linked to more severe reactions, most likely because the lung is more vulnerable to wheezing symptoms during a food-allergic reaction.

How many people die from food allergies?

We do not have exact numbers, but it appears to be uncommon. Some researchers have calculated that more people die from lightning strikes. But fatalities do occur, most often striking teenagers and young adults. It is important to realize that these tragedies are preventable. Avoiding severe and fatal allergic reactions to foods requires education about avoidance and knowing how and when to treat an allergic reaction.

When Symptoms Are Not a Food Allergy

What common medical problems do people wrongly attribute to food allergy?

Various maladies have been attributed to food allergies despite the link being unproven or even being disproven. Symptoms and illnesses with which a relationship to food allergy remains controversial or unproven include behavioral and developmental problems in children, headaches, and weight gain. Some illnesses that are attributed to food "allergy" may actually be triggered by the chemical components of the foods, not really an allergy. Additionally, allergic symptoms are sometimes wrongly attributed to foods when a different allergic cause is the culprit.

What are examples of allergic conditions that can be wrongly attributed to a food allergy?

Food and nonfood triggers of allergic symptoms can cause the same symptoms, which can lead to confusion. For example, hives can be triggered by a virus. Wheezing and nasal symptoms of itching, sneezing, and congestion are often triggered by allergens in the air, such as pollens or animal dander. Chronic rashes can be triggered by irritants such as soaps, infections, sweating, or allergens in the air.

Can foods affect behavior?

Possibly, but not typically through allergy. Caffeine in foods may cause irritability or increased activity because of a pharmacologic (drug) effect. Sugar does not appear to affect behavior. Some studies support the notion that chemical colors and preservatives adversely affect some children's attention or trigger hyperactivity, but this is not attributed to allergy. Rather, the connection is purported to be caused by the chemical effects of these additives. If a true food allergy affected behavior, it would likely do so only indirectly, such as through chronic disruptive symptoms, like itchy rashes, that interrupt sleep.

Can foods cause headaches (migraine)?

Possibly, but not through allergy. Chemicals in some foods, such as fermented foods and hard cheeses, may trigger migraines in some people, but this is not an allergic reaction. Some of the additional foods considered triggers for migraine include alcoholic beverages, banana, caffeine (withdrawal or too much), chocolate, monosodium glutamate, nitrites and nitrates, nuts, and seeds.

Can a food allergy cause weight gain?

This is a common misconception, especially attributed to wheat. Severe allergies are more likely to cause weight loss or poor weight gain because the gut does not respond properly. Cakes and cookies may result in weight gain, but this is because of their calories, not an allergy!

Can food allergy cause fatigue?

Not specifically. However, a person with chronic malnutrition and allergic symptoms due to food allergies may become fatigued from the illnesses.

Masqueraders of Food Allergy

In what ways might symptoms masquerade as a possible food allergy?
The symptoms of food allergy—in the skin, the gut, breathing, and other places—are also the symptoms of many other medical problems. We eat food and snacks throughout the day, and it is natural to wonder whether food is triggering a variety of symptoms. For example, a rash could be an allergy to a trigger other than food, or it could have no relationship to either food or allergies (for example, viral illnesses, autoimmune diseases like arthritis, or blood diseases such as porphyria all can result in skin rashes). In this section I focus on common "mimics" of food allergy.

I have trouble breathing, develop tingling and numbness in my fingers, and feel light-headed. Is this a food allergy?
This group of symptoms certainly shares some features with an allergic reaction. But these are also common symptoms of breathing quickly and deeply, a problem called hyperventilation.

How does hyperventilation mimic a food allergy?
When a person hyperventilates, such as from anxiety, changes in the chemicals in the bloodstream can cause symptoms. Light-headedness, difficulty breathing, and general discomfort are similar to symptoms of a food-allergic reaction. Calming down and breathing into a bag should help. This situation can mimic a food-allergic reaction, especially if a person is concerned about possible exposure to an allergenic food, which leads to anxiety and possible hyperventilation.

I notice blistering and burning on my skin in the summer when I have gin and tonic. Is that an allergy?
The sun and the lime juice, not an allergy, are causing the blistering and burning. There are chemicals in limes, lemons, celery, parsnips, and parsley that are called psoralens. When these chemicals are on the skin and exposed to the sun, a reaction may occur that results in a burn, with blistering and redness over the next few days. This may occur on the hands of people preparing the drinks or foods or on the lips of those eating or drinking the foods. To avoid this reaction, wash off the juices right away and avoid the sun when working with or ingesting foods with psoralens in them.

My nose runs after eating hot or spicy foods. Is that an allergy?

The chemical that makes some foods hot or spicy can also trigger a runny nose through a neurologic response. Some people are more sensitive to this than others. Sometimes the temperature of a food—for example, steaming hot beverages or soups—will trigger runny nose symptoms, again based on neurologic, not allergic, responses.

I often sneeze while eating breakfast, no matter what the food. Is this an allergy?

There are many triggers of sneezing in the morning. A buildup of mucus from the night before can trigger a sneeze. Another cause of morning sneezing is sunlight. As the sun flickers through the window, it can trigger a neurologic response in some people that makes them sneeze.

When I ate fish, I had allergic symptoms, but so did others at the table. Is that an allergy?

This description fits scombroid fish poisoning. When dark-meat fish like tuna or mahi-mahi spoils, it can develop histamine-like toxins. Histamine is the chemical made by allergy cells that cause allergic symptoms. When the histamine-like toxin from the spoiled fish is eaten, a person may experience symptoms of mouth and throat itching, stomach pain, and skin redness that fully mimic an allergic reaction.

My child develops a red streak on her face when she eats certain foods. Is that an allergy?

If there is no swelling or itching, and the red streak always develops in the same area, it may be something called auriculotemporal syndrome, also known as Frey syndrome or gustatory flushing. The streak runs from the corner of the mouth to the ear on one side of the face when a tart-tasting food promotes salivation; the streak is the result of minor nerve damage.

I experience episodes of hives and diarrhea, episodes of itch and flushing, and sometimes it occurs with meals. My doctor says I have mast cell activation syndrome. Is it a food allergy?

Mast cell activation syndrome (MCAS) is a medical problem where cells called mast cells release chemicals like histamine in large amounts from minor triggers. The resulting symptoms are like those of any allergic reaction. It is diagnosed by a full medical evaluation that shows inappropriate levels of the chemical released by these cells, along with typical symptom patterns. People with MCAS do not necessarily have any food allergies. Many things may trigger reactions, however, including stress, aspirin-type medications, narcotic-type medications, extreme temperatures, and insect stings. Food allergy per se is not a trigger (although a person with MCAS can have food allergy), but alcohol and spicy foods may be triggers in some people.

Prevalence of Food Allergies

How common are food allergies?

Estimates vary globally and regionally, but more than 1% and less than 10% of the population is estimated to have food allergies, with 4% to 10% of children and 3% to 10% of adults affected.

Is there really an increase in food allergies, or is there just more awareness or publicity?

Several studies support the conclusions of most experts that there truly has been an increase over the past few decades. Studies that I have been involved in suggest a tripling in peanut allergy among children between 1997 and 2008, now with more than 1 in 70 children affected in some areas of the United States.

Why does one person develop a food allergy and another does not?

Genetic predisposition (allergies run in families) and environmental factors (exposure to foods, components of the diet, and other factors) play a role.

Why would the body attack foods if it only results in damage and bad reactions?

I agree that no obvious good comes from having food allergies. One theory is that the attack on foods is a misdirected one. The part of the immune system that is activated against proteins in foods is the same part that fights parasite, or worm, infections. Perhaps persons who develop allergies would be well protected if they lived in a setting with parasites, but otherwise their immune system response to harmless proteins, such as those in foods, is counterproductive.

Causes and Triggers of Food Allergies

What foods cause food allergies?
Any food. More than 170 foods have been noted to cause a reaction.

What are the most common foods to trigger allergies?
Milk, eggs, peanuts, tree nuts, shellfish, fish, wheat, and soy account for the most significant allergies. Allergies to fruits and vegetables are usually less severe. Allergies to seeds, such as sesame, are being increasingly reported.

Aren't chocolate, corn, strawberries, and tomatoes common food allergens?
These foods have been frequently listed as common allergens, but studies do not identify them as such. There are definitely true allergies to these four foods. But people may experience problems with these foods because some of them have chemicals with irritant properties that cause mild allergy-like symptoms. These reactions are often inconsistent, and a person may have mild symptoms only sometimes when eating the food.

Do children have different food allergy triggers than adults?
Children are more likely to have allergies to egg, milk, soy, and wheat. These are less common allergens in adults, partly because they are usually outgrown during childhood. Infants and young children are not likely to have developed allergies related to raw fruits and vegetables because these are pollen-related allergies (see the discussion of oral allergy syndrome earlier in this chapter), and people typically have to experience a few pollen seasons to become allergic.

Can a person be allergic to fats?
No. A person may have trouble digesting fats, however.

Can a person be allergic to sugars?
Not to simple sugars like those found in most foods.

Can a person be allergic to iodide?
No. There is a misconception that an "iodide allergy" is at the root of both

seafood allergies and allergies to injected dyes used for radiographic medical tests. However, iodide does not trigger typical allergic reactions such as hives, wheezing, or anaphylaxis. In fact, iodide is in salt, which we all eat.

If I am allergic to one food, does that mean I will be allergic to related foods?

The answer depends on the food or food group. Table 1.4 gives general rates of allergy to related foods. You should talk about your concerns of allergy to related foods with your allergist. In general, allergy tests overestimate allergy to related foods and can be misleading. It concerns me when a person stops eating a tolerated food just because they developed an allergy to a related food (for example, it is not necessary to stop eating tolerated beans because of a peanut allergy even though peanut is a legume [bean]). Table 1.4 shows approximate rates of cross-reactivity. There is a difference between having allergy to related foods because of similar proteins in the foods (cross-reactivity) and allergy that happens to coexist because people with a genetic disposition toward food allergy tend to be allergic to multiple foods, and they tend to be common allergens. An example of the latter is that about a third of people with peanut allergy are allergic to at least one type of tree nut, but peanut (a bean) and tree nuts are not closely related botanically.

If a food is organic or farm-raised, does that change the allergic potential?

No. The proteins are the same.

Does cooking a food make it less allergenic?

The answer depends on the food and how it is heated. Some foods appear to become more likely to trigger an allergic reaction (increased allergenicity) when heated. For example, dry-roasting peanuts appears to make the proteins more capable of triggering an allergic response, while boiling peanuts does not have that effect. Heating fruits and vegetables usually makes them less allergenic for people with protein-induced food allergies. Boiling milk does not appear to significantly change its allergenic properties, but heating it to high temperatures (in an oven) in the "airy" environment of a cake alters some of the proteins, reducing their allergenicity.

What do I need to know about allergies to specific foods?

When you know you have an allergy to a food, you need to know whether to worry about related foods as described above. Understanding some features of certain foods can help you better understand potential risk of allergy and how to avoid reactions. The questions and answers that follow address major food allergens, common food groups, and food additives.

Table 1.4. Approximate Rates of Allergy to Related Foods

Primary Food	Cross-Reaction Rate	More Details
Finned bony fish (cod, salmon, tuna)	Other finned fish: 50%	Cartilaginous fish (ray, shark dogfish): under 5%
Crustacean shellfish (crab, lobster, shrimp)	Other crustacean: 75%	Bivalves and mollusks (clam, mussel, squid): under 50%
Bivalves and mollusks (clam, mussel, squid)	Crustaceans: over 70%	
Cow's milk	Goat and sheep: over 90%	Camel and mare: under 5% Beef: 10% to 20%
Wheat	Barley and rye: under 25%	
Peanut	Legumes overall: 5% to 10%	Green bean, pea, soy: 5% to 20% Lupine: 20% Sesame: 10% to 15% (co-allergy) Tree nut: 33% (co-allergy)
Soy	Peanut: over 75%	
Chickpea	Lentil, pea: over 50%	
Tree nut	Another tree nut: 15% to 33%	If walnut: 66% pecan If pecan: over 95% walnut If cashew: 66% pistachio If pistachio: over 95% cashew
Sesame	Other seeds: low risk	

Peanuts

What kind of food are peanuts?
They are beans (legumes).

Do any foods have increased risks of allergy for people with a peanut allergy?
Children with a peanut allergy have a higher risk of having other food allergies, not necessarily only because of similarities in proteins among foods (peanut is a bean) but also because of a general disposition toward food allergy. For example, egg and peanut are unrelated, but having an allergy to one is a risk for allergy to the other.

What foods might have peanuts in them?
Peanuts are everywhere. They are found in many manufactured products, such as baked goods, candy, chocolate, and ice cream. Ethnic restaurants (such as African, Chinese, Indonesian, Thai, and Vietnamese), bakeries, and ice cream parlors use peanut products in many foods. Peanut butter or peanut flour may be used as a "secret" ingredient to thicken and flavor chili and spaghetti sauce.

Are peanuts used in nonfood items?
Yes. Peanuts may be found in cosmetics, medicines, nutritional supplements, and pet foods, for example.

Is peanut oil safe for a person with peanut allergy?
It may be, but I advise against routinely using peanut oil. Peanut protein is found in unrefined peanut oils that are cold-pressed, expelled, expressed, and extruded from peanut. These oils are unsafe. Highly refined peanut oils contain only the leftover fat after the protein is removed. These oils should be safe, but it may be difficult to identify the type of oil used in a product. Therefore I recommend avoiding peanut oil or taking extreme care to ensure the safe peanut oil is used.

Can a person with a peanut allergy eat tree nuts?
No significant proteins are similar between peanut and tree nuts. Although

most people with a peanut allergy will tolerate some or all tree nuts, many tree nuts (such as almonds, pecans, walnuts, etc.) are processed with peanuts and therefore may contain trace amounts of peanut protein, making these foods risky. Candies and chocolates also are often processed with peanuts. Therefore, for practical purposes, many individuals and families choose to avoid tree nuts and most candy and chocolate when there is a peanut allergy. Options for eating tree nuts despite having a peanut allergy are discussed further in chapter 6.

Eggs

Are people allergic to the egg white or yolk?

The proteins most likely to cause allergic reactions are found in the white. But most allergists suggest avoiding both the white and the yolk because it is difficult to separate these components in cooking.

If I am allergic to chicken eggs, do I need to avoid other types of eggs?

Yes. People with chicken egg allergy are likely to be allergic to other poultry eggs, like quail.

Does having a chicken egg allergy mean that I would be allergic to fish eggs?

No.

Can people with an egg allergy eat foods that have eggs baked into them, such as muffins or waffles?

About 70% of people with an egg allergy can tolerate small amounts of egg in baked goods like cookies.

Why can some people with an egg allergy eat eggs in baked forms?

The process of heating the egg in a bakery food that rises and develops air cells allows the egg protein to get superheated and alters the proteins. For some people, this is enough to make the food safe to eat. This is different than simply baking an egg. There may also be a difference in the amount of egg being consumed, with baked goods having less.

If I am allergic to eggs and have not tried to eat eggs in baked goods, can I try these foods?

No. You need to discuss this with your allergist. A severe reaction is possible (unless you are already eating those products successfully).

What words or ingredients might indicate that a food contains eggs?

US labeling laws require use of the word "egg" on product ingredient labels. Words that may refer to eggs as ingredients are albumin, egg (dried, lecithin, powdered, solids, white, yolk), eggnog, globulin, lysozyme (used in Europe), mayonnaise, meringue, ovalbumin, and ovovitellin.

What foods might have eggs in them?

Eggs may be found in baked goods, breaded foods, candies, canned soups, casseroles, cream fillings, custards, eggnog, frostings, ice creams, lollipops, marshmallows, marzipan, meat-based dishes such as meatballs or meatloaf, nougat, pastas, and salad dressings. Egg whites and shells may be used as clarifying agents in coffees, consommés, bouillons, soup stocks, and wines. A shiny glaze on baked goods may be an "egg wash."

Can I use an egg replacer or egg substitute if I have an egg allergy?

Be careful! Don't get tricked. Most "egg substitutes" contain eggs.

Are eggs used in nonfood items?

Yes. Eggs may be found in cosmetics, medicines, nutritional supplements, and pet foods.

What vaccines have egg in them?

There is not enough egg in the measles, mumps, and rubella (MMR) vaccine to cause an allergic reaction. Therefore this vaccine poses no greater risk to people with an egg allergy than it does to people without one. Some forms of the yearly influenza vaccine have traces of egg protein, but people with egg allergy are advised to get the immunization anyway, because studies have shown no increased risks. Ask your doctor. People traveling to areas where contracting yellow fever is a risk might need a vaccine that contains egg. A person with an egg allergy would need to be given this vaccine only under special circumstances by an allergist.

What medications have egg in them?
An anesthetic agent called propofol has a fatty derivative from eggs; the medical literature is unclear on whether this is a risk, but so far it appears unlikely. Otherwise, egg is not a common ingredient in medications, but it is prudent to check any medication for inclusion of food allergens.

Cow's Milk

What proteins in milk cause milk allergies?
Milk contains many proteins, including casein and whey. The casein proteins appear to be the most potent allergens, but often a person with a milk allergy reacts to many of the proteins in milk. Even if whey proteins are tolerated, most foods with milk in them, including those listing only whey ingredients, contain some amount of casein as well.

Are other foods a concern for a person with a milk allergy?
Among people with severe cow's milk allergy, about 10% may react to beef, especially if it is rare, because some proteins that cause allergy in some people are in both the cow's milk and blood.

Can people with a milk allergy eat foods that have milk baked into them, such as muffins, or can they tolerate some cheeses?
About 70% of people with milk allergy can tolerate smaller amounts of milk in baked goods like cookies. Some people can even tolerate well-heated cheese.

Why can some people with a milk allergy eat milk in baked forms?
The process of heating the milk in the "airy" environment of a baked good alters the proteins. For some people, this is enough to make the food safe to eat. These effects do not occur when simply heating a glass of milk.

If I am allergic to milk and have not tried to eat milk in baked goods, or cheese, can I try these foods?
No. You need to discuss this with your allergist. A severe reaction is possible (unless you are already eating those products successfully).

What terms might indicate that a food contains milk or is a dairy food?
US labeling laws require that the term "milk" be used if it is an ingredient.
Milk shows up in all sorts of foods, so watch out for artificial butter flavor,
butter, butter fat, butter oil, casein and caseinates (in all forms), cheese (all
types), cheese flavor, cream, curds, custard, ghee, hydrolysates (casein, milk
protein, protein, whey, whey protein), ice cream, lactalbumin, lactalbumin
phosphate, lactoferrin, lactoglobulin, lactulose, nougat, pudding, Recaldent
(used in teeth-whitening chewing gums), rennet, rennet casein, Simplesse,
whey (in all forms), and yogurt. Milk can be found in breads, cakes, caramels,
cereals, chewing gum, chocolates, cold cuts, cookies, crackers, margarines,
nondairy products, processed and canned meats, and refrigerated and frozen
soy products.

If a food is labeled "kosher pareve (or parve)," is it milk-free?
Just because a product is kosher, to be eaten as "nondairy" (pareve or parve),
does not mean it doesn't have some milk protein. In kosher labeling, a D on a
product label next to the circled K or U indicates the presence of milk protein.

**Does "nondairy" on a label mean the food is safe for people with a
milk allergy?**
No. Some products, such as nondairy creamers, contain milk ingredients.
The label should include the term "milk," but seeing "nondairy" could be
misleading. This is an example of why reading the entire ingredient label
is necessary to avoid trouble.

**What are some unexpected places where milk might be an ingredient
or a contaminant?**
Milk may be found in cosmetics, medicines, nutritional supplements, and
pet foods. Deli meats could become contaminated with milk from cheeses
cut on the same slicer. Sometimes fish or shellfish are "dunked" in milk
or have milk protein added to reduce odors or change the consistency, so
watch out for this practice and choose fresh forms.

Do lactose-containing foods or medicines have milk protein in them?
Lactose is milk sugar and is not an allergen (not a protein). But it is derived
from milk. There are rare reports of lactose products triggering reactions
in persons with milk allergy. In particular, residual milk protein in lactose
used in some types of asthma inhalers, in some injected steroid formula-

tions, and in preparations used to measure lactose intolerance triggered symptoms in extremely sensitive milk-allergic people.

If I have a milk allergy, can I use a medication in pill form that has lactose in it?

Pharmaceutical-grade lactose in oral medications has not triggered significant reports of reactions, possibly indicating a very low risk. It seems that lactose is usually free of milk proteins but may sometimes have a trace amount. If you wish to avoid the risk of trace contamination, formulations without lactose are usually possible to obtain. Often, the liquid forms are lactose-free. You should investigate products individually and speak with your allergist about the risks.

Does cocoa butter or calcium lactate have milk?

You do not usually need to worry about calcium lactate, cocoa butter, coconut milk, cream of tartar, or oleoresin.

Is dark chocolate or cocoa safe for a person with a milk allergy?

Cocoa is a bean and a very uncommon allergen. Pure cocoa is safe for people with a milk allergy. Milk chocolate is clearly a problem for a person with a milk allergy, but many dark chocolates do not have milk ingredients and could be safe. However, studies have shown a high rate of milk contamination in dark chocolate candy products, even some without advisory labeling ("may contain milk"). Therefore I advise caution. Chocolates may be better purchased from specialty manufacturers that cater to people with food allergies (see the resources in chapter 11).

What formulas can be given to a baby with milk allergy?

More than 90% of infants with milk allergy tolerate formulas approved as "hypoallergenic," specifically a type called an extensive casein hydrolysate. The formula is made of digested cow's milk protein. Most infants with cow's milk allergy will also tolerate soy, which has no relation to cow's milk but is in itself somewhat allergenic. A partially digested cow's milk–based formula, such as a partial whey hydrolysate, would not be a good choice because residual milk protein can trigger a reaction. If a hypoallergenic formula is not tolerated, a formula made from the building blocks of protein, amino acids, could be used. This type of formula, called an elemental formula, or amino acid–based formula, is expensive and poor-tasting.

Wheat and Other Grains

Is wheat allergy the same as celiac disease?

Wheat allergy is different from celiac disease (also called sprue, or gluten-sensitive enteropathy). This is discussed more in chapter 5.

If I have a wheat allergy, what other grains can I eat?

Most people with a wheat allergy (about 80%) can tolerate other grains, such as barley and rye, but wheat contamination of other grains is sometimes a problem. Although you may need to check with your doctor before trying one, flour substitutes that are usually less allergenic include those made from amaranth, arrowroot, barley, buckwheat (which is not a type of wheat), corn, millet, oat, potato, quinoa, rice, soybean, and tapioca.

What terms on a label might indicate wheat, and what types of foods are often made of wheat?

Ingredients and foods of concern include breadcrumbs, bulgur, cereal extract, couscous, durum (durum flour or wheat), einkorn, emmer, farina, flour (all-purpose, cake, enriched, graham, high-gluten, high-protein, pastry, wheat), Kamut (khorasan), semolina, spelt, sprouted wheat, triticale, vital gluten, wheat (bran, germ, gluten, malt, starch), and whole wheat berries. Expect to find wheat in ale, baked products, baking mixes, batter-fried foods, beer, breaded foods, breakfast cereals, candy, crackers, frankfurters and other processed meats, ice cream products, salad dressings, sauces, soups, soy sauce, and surimi.

What do I need to know about allergies to other grains?

Although it is possible to be allergic to any of the numerous grains and grain substitutes (amaranth, arrowroot, barley, buckwheat, corn, millet, oat, potato, quinoa, and rice), these are uncommon allergies. Those who are allergic to corn can usually have corn oil and corn syrup because they are not likely to have relevant amounts of protein.

Can a wheat-allergic person safely eat a communion wafer?

No. The wheat could trigger a reaction.

What communion wafer substitutes are available for a person with a wheat allergy?

For someone with a true wheat allergy, an entirely wheat-free substitute (such as a rice-based wafer) would be the safest option. There is a low-gluten communion wafer, acceptable to the Vatican, for Catholics with celiac disease. The gluten content is 0.01%, which comes to 37 micrograms of gluten. The trace amount of wheat protein in the low-gluten formulation carries a very small risk of inducing a reaction in a highly sensitive wheat-allergic person. Most people with a wheat allergy would be able to tolerate this low amount, however, assuming the wheat content is accurate. A person could work with an allergist to determine through past reactions and possibly a medically supervised feeding whether the wafer would be safe. You should also check the full ingredients list for other allergens you are avoiding.

Tree Nuts

What foods are tree nuts?

The US Food and Drug Administration (FDA) considers *a lot* of foods to be nuts. The main ones are almonds, Brazil nuts, cashews, chestnuts, coconuts, filberts (hazelnuts), macadamias, pecans, pine nuts (pignolia nuts), pistachios, and walnuts. For pictures of peanut and common nuts, see figure 1.1.

Are people with a tree nut allergy also allergic to peanuts?

People who are allergic to tree nuts are not necessarily allergic to peanuts (or vice versa), although there is increased risk because nuts are all more allergenic foods.

If you are allergic to one tree nut, are you allergic to all tree nuts?

People can be allergic to some tree nuts and not others, for example, allergic to walnuts but not cashews or almonds. But some nuts have similar proteins—almonds and hazelnuts, pistachios and cashews, walnuts and pecans. A person often has an allergy to both. See table 1.4.

What is the relationship between cashews, mangoes, and pink peppercorns?

These three foods are from the same food family (Anacardiaceae). The mango pit is allergenic, but not the pulp, which is the edible part. Therefore having a cashew allergy does not mean there will be a problem eating mango pulp, although it is possible to be allergic to that part of the mango as well. Pink peppercorns (also known as Brazilian pepper, Christmas berry, Rose pepper, and others) are also related to cashew and may be a risk. Pink peppercorns are different from other peppers (bell peppers, "chili" peppers, green peppers, and others). The dried berry may be used as a spice, although its use is not currently widespread. There have been rare reports of allergic reactions to citrus fruit seeds and to pectin in people with severe cashew allergy.

Is coconut a tree nut?

The FDA considers it a nut, but there is controversy. Most people consider coconut to be a fruit (a fibrous, one-seeded drupe).

If I have a tree nut allergy, can I eat coconut?

Coconut allergy is uncommon. Some coconut proteins are similar to those in walnuts, hazelnuts, lentils, and other foods, yet most people with allergies to these foods tolerate coconut. There are relatively few reports of coconut allergy in the literature, even among those with tree nut allergies. This is a situation where you should talk to your doctor unless you are already tolerating coconut. Coconut oil, probably containing little coconut protein to begin with, is a low risk.

Is shea nut butter an allergen?

So far, no allergic reactions to shea nut butter have been documented in the literature. In at least one study, no proteins could be detected in this derivative of shea nuts.

Is lychee (lichee) a nut?

The FDA has included lychee on its list of "nuts" that require labeling disclosure, but it is actually a tropical and subtropical fruit. It is sometimes referred to as a "nut" when eaten in its dried form. Lychee is a rare allergen, but like most foods, it has been reported to cause a severe allergic reaction in a few people. It has some allergenic relationships with latex, pollens, and sunflower seeds.

What foods might have nut ingredients?

Labeling laws require that a tree nut ingredient be named. Tree nut avoidance can be tricky because the nuts can be found in barbeque sauces, candies, cereals, chocolates, some cold cuts (such as mortadella), cookies, crackers, energy bars, flavored coffees, frozen desserts, gianduja (a creamy mixture of chocolate and chopped almonds and hazelnuts, although other nuts may be used), marinades, marzipan (almond paste), nougat, Nu-Nuts artificial nuts, Nutella, nut meal, and pesto. Some alcoholic beverages may contain nut flavorings. Natural extracts such as pure almond and wintergreen may have nut proteins (which could trigger a filbert/hazelnut allergy).

Which cuisines typically use tree nuts?

Tree nuts are common ingredients in foods from bakeries, ethnic restaurants (such as African, Chinese, Indian, Thai, and Vietnamese), and ice cream parlors.

What nonfood items could have tree nut ingredients?

Tree nut oils may be found in cosmetics, lotions and soaps, medications, nutritional supplements, and pet foods. Acorns are probably allergenic, but they are too sour for us to eat, so we will leave them for the squirrels.

Can I have artificial nut flavor if I am nut allergic?

Imitation and artificially flavored extracts are generally safe.

Is almond extract safe with an almond allergy?

Pure almond extract should be avoided because it likely has almond proteins. Peach or apricot pit extracts may also be used for making almond extract. Artificial and imitation almond extracts should be safe, although contacting the manufacturer is advisable. Alternatively, a different flavor, such as vanilla, could be substituted.

Can I have nut oils if I am allergic to tree nuts?

There can be a risk in eating these. Nut oils are not generally refined, so they do contain tree nut proteins.

Can I have butternut squash, nutmeg, and water chestnuts if I have a nut allergy?

Although butternut squash, nutmeg, and water chestnuts have the word "nut" in them, they are not peanuts or tree nuts. Nutmeg contains a chemical called myristicin, which in large amounts can induce dangerous toxic effects and hallucinations. Although donuts also have the word "nut" in them, you will need to consider the exact ingredients to know if they really have any tree nuts in them!

If I am allergic to one nut, do I need to avoid all nuts?

A person may be allergic to one or two or many nuts. Avoiding all nuts when there is an allergy to just one or two is a personal decision.

What are the risks of eating other nuts when there are allergies to some?

The risks include:

- making a mistake in identification and eating the allergenic nuts
- getting exposed to the avoided nuts because of cross-contact with the nuts that are safe (if a walnut brownie also has cashews or pistachios, for example)

How often do allergies develop to a nut that is already tolerated?

If a nut is already tolerated as a routine part of the diet, developing a new allergy to it is uncommon. A new nut allergy can occur at any age, however.

What considerations are important in deciding whether to eat some types of nuts when there are allergies to other types?

Some people decide to avoid all nuts to reduce their risk of accidentally eating the ones they are avoiding. Others choose to eat the tolerated nuts, being careful about the foods they select. Because nuts are often processed together, it is difficult to find ones that are not at risk for cross-contact. Almonds are often selected as a tolerated nut to try because they can be purchased in various forms without contamination by other nuts. For example, specific brands of almond butter, almond milk, and cereals are not processed with other nuts. The decision to eat some nuts should be discussed with your doctor, for it involves considering risks (severity of allergy), dietary preferences, age, and other factors. Knowing what nuts look like is important in making these decisions. Pictures of nuts are shown in figure 1.1.

Can a person with a nut allergy eat hickory-smoked foods?

Hickory smoking uses the wood from the hickory tree, not the nuts, and so there should be no risk.

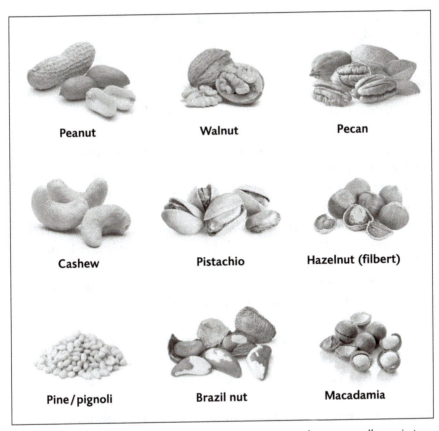

Peanut   **Walnut**   **Pecan**

Cashew   **Pistachio**   **Hazelnut (filbert)**

Pine/pignoli   **Brazil nut**   **Macadamia**

Figure 1.1. Shown here to aid identification are peanut and common allergenic tree nuts.

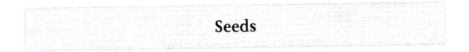

Seeds

What are examples of seeds?

There are many kinds of seeds, including flax, mustard, poppy, pumpkin, sesame, sunflower, and others.

If I am allergic to one seed, am I allergic to all seeds?

Allergy to one seed does not necessarily mean allergy to others.

Is it possible to tolerate eating a few seeds when eating more of that seed can trigger a reaction?

Yes. Since seeds are often used in small amounts in foods, people with seed allergies may have no problems because they never eat enough to cause symptoms. For example, sesame seeds on breads might be tolerated, but tahini, a paste that is primarily sesame protein, may trigger a reaction.

If I tolerate some sesame seeds on bread but react to larger amounts in tahini, do I need to avoid sesame on breads?

There are several issues to consider here. If a reaction to tahini was severe, you may be more motivated to completely avoid sesame in any form. If you routinely tolerate stray seeds, allowing them to remain in your diet may be less concerning. We do not know if eating a few seeds speeds, hinders, or has no effect on recovery from the allergy. A compromise may include not worrying about stray seeds but avoiding larger amounts. Such decisions should be made in consultation with your allergist.

Which seeds are most likely to cause allergy?

Sesame allergy is the most common seed allergy. Mustard and poppy seeds can also cause allergies, but these are comparatively uncommon.

If I have a sesame allergy, do I need to worry about allergies to other foods?

Sesame, like most foods, shares some proteins with other plants. For example, there is some relationship to peanuts, although most people with a peanut allergy tolerate sesame.

What products or ingredients may have sesame?

Sesame was added to US labeling laws in 2021, with an effective date of January 1, 2023, requiring labels to disclose this ingredient. Other seeds are not currently included in US labeling laws. Food ingredients that indicate the presence of sesame include benne, sesame flour, sesame oil, sesame seed, tahini (sesame paste), and til or teel. Sesame is often in bagels, baked goods, breadcrumbs, breads, breakfast cereals (such as granola, muesli, and Kashi brand cereals), crackers, dipping sauces and marinades, dips such as hummus and baba ghanoush, falafel, halvah, Japanese snack mix, protein and energy bars, rolls, sushi, tortilla chips, vegetarian "burgers," and herbal drinks, including Aqua Libra, a British herbal beverage.

Is sesame found in nonfood items?

Sesame may be found in cosmetics, medications, nutritional supplements, and pet foods. The scientific name for sesame, *Sesamum indicum*, might be on the label.

Is sesame oil safe for people with sesame allergies?

Sesame oil is usually not refined and therefore contains sesame proteins, so it is not safe.

Soy

If I have a soy allergy, can I eat peanuts and other beans?

Soy is a bean, yet most people with a peanut allergy are not allergic to soy. People with a soy allergy may be able to eat peanuts too, although the risk of being allergic to peanuts is increased if you are already allergic to soy.

What foods or terms on labels indicate soy?

Labeling laws require use of the term "soy" if it is an ingredient. Foods and words to look out for include edamame, miso, natto, shoyu sauce, soy (fiber, flour, grits, nuts, sprouts), soy protein (concentrate, hydrolyzed, isolate), soy sauce, soy substitutes (cheese, ice cream, milk, yogurt), tamari, tempeh, textured (or texturized) vegetable protein (TVP), and tofu (soybean curd). Soy is in many foods to add protein, such as baking mixes, breads, breakfast cereals, canned broths and soups, canned tuna and meat, cookies, crackers, high-protein energy bars and snacks, low-fat peanut butters, and processed meat, such as frankfurters. Eating at Asian restaurants is risky because soy is a frequent ingredient. Highly refined soy oil has no appreciable residual protein and is exempt from labeling, but it is often included on ingredient labels anyway.

Is soy found in nonfood items?

Soy may be found in cosmetics, medications, nutritional supplements, and pet foods.

Is it possible to tolerate soy but have reactions to soy protein isolate?

Yes. Soy protein isolate (also referred to as soy protein concentrate) may have a concentrated amount of a particular protein from soy that is more allergenic for some people.

If I have reacted to soy protein isolate, do I need to avoid all soy?

The exact risks vary from person to person. Many people who react to soy protein isolate appear to tolerate other forms of soy, for example, soy flour in bread. It is often reasonable to continue eating the tolerated forms. Your individual circumstances, particularly the severity of past reactions, should be discussed with an allergist. Soy protein isolate may be found in hamburgers, health bars, health food drinks, soups, and various other foods.

If I have a soy allergy, can I eat soy oil?

Yes. Soy oil is refined and is generally considered safe for people with soy allergy.

If I have a soy allergy, can I eat soy lecithin?

Most people with a soy allergy will tolerate foods that contain soy lecithin. This fatty derivative of soy has minimal protein and is used in low amounts in foods, often simply as a nonstick agent in baking.

I have a soy allergy, but I am able to eat soy sauce. Why would that be?

Soy sauce is the product of fermentation, and very little soy protein is left intact in soy sauce.

Legumes

What do I need to know about allergy to beans?

Among the numerous types of beans, peanuts and soybeans are the most common allergens. Allergies to chickpeas and lentils are more common in Mediterranean countries.

If I am allergic to one bean, do I need to avoid all beans?

Usually not. It seems that, among beans, peanuts and soy are the main culprits. There is a bean called lupine (lupin) that may be higher on the problem list than others, especially if someone already has a peanut allergy. Next in line are lentils, chickpeas, and green peas. Allergy to kidney beans, lima beans, navy beans, string beans, and others are far less common. A person with an allergy to one bean can usually eat other beans, but a person who has had reactions to several beans might have trouble with most beans.

I tolerate canned beans but have reactions to raw ones. How is this possible?

Sometimes people are sensitive to pollen-related proteins in beans, which are destroyed by cooking or canning.

I tolerate peas, but I had an allergic reaction to pea soup. How is this possible?

The amount of protein is much higher in pea soup than in separate peas, for example, peas and carrots or a serving of peas on a plate. People with an allergy may have a threshold beyond which they begin to have allergic reactions. They may tolerate soybeans (edamame) but not soy milk or products with concentrated soy protein (soy protein concentrate/soy protein isolate). They may tolerate chickpeas on a salad but not a serving of hummus. They may tolerate lentils on a salad but not lentil soup. Many products are using concentrated bean proteins as a protein substitute, which can be tricky and risky for people with a bean allergy.

What types of products have concentrated bean proteins and could be a problem for those with bean allergies?

As mentioned above, some sources of concentrated bean protein are obvious, such as pea soup, lentil soup, or soy milk. However, soy protein isolate/concentrate may be added to energy bars, soups, and other processed foods. Flours in breads and pastas may substitute lentil, lupine or chickpea. Concentrated pea proteins (especially using yellow peas, also called dun peas) may be used to fortify meat substitutes, processed meats, yogurts, cookies, and various health supplements. These products may tout the ingredients with words such as hydrolyzed pea protein, pea fiber, pea protein, or pea protein isolate.

What is lupine?

Lupine, also called lupin, is a type of bean that can be found in many gluten-free, high-protein, and specialty food products, such as pastas and breads. In parts of Europe and Australia, lupine flour is often mixed with wheat flour in baked goods.

Are there hidden sources of legumes?

Legumes can be dried and used as a flour. Some pastas are fortified with beans such as chickpeas, lentils, or lupines.

Vegetables and Starches

What do I need to know about allergies to vegetables?

Countless vegetables have various botanical relationships to each other and to pollens. Many allergic reactions to vegetables are related to pollen allergies. People with allergies to pollen may have mild allergic reactions to raw forms of a vegetable that has similar proteins to those in the pollen (see the discussion of pollen-associated food allergy syndrome earlier in this chapter). Symptoms often vary depending on whether the food is cooked, which makes a reaction less likely to occur. Not all vegetable allergies can be tied to pollen allergies, however. People have also reported mild and, rarely, severe reactions to many vegetables without a clear connection to pollen allergies. Some of the more common culprits appear to be carrot, celery, and eggplant (which is actually a fruit).

Are some vegetables more allergenic than others?

It is difficult to find reports of allergies to artichokes, asparagus, broccoli, Brussels sprouts, cabbage, cauliflower, lettuce, mushrooms (fungus), olives, squash, or sweet potatoes. Many other vegetables are more problematic than these, but reactions are still relatively uncommon. It is thought that some reactions, such as those to eggplant, may be caused by natural chemicals in the food that trigger allergy-like symptoms.

I can eat baked potatoes and French fries, but I sometimes get itchy from potato salad. Is that a sign of potato allergy?

Sometimes the potatoes used in potato salad are less cooked than other forms. Raw potatoes have residual proteins similar to those in birch pollens, whereas these proteins are destroyed when potatoes are cooked. In this case, the reaction may be to these proteins, assuming there is no allergy to other ingredients in the potato salad.

Fruits

What fruits can cause allergic reactions?

There are countless fruits (berries, citrus, melons, pitted fruits, and so on) with many botanical relationships, and virtually all have caused a reaction in someone.

Are fruit allergies severe?

Most allergies to fruits are mild. Many reactions to fruits are related to a person having allergies to pollens and then experiencing mild allergic reactions, such as an itchy mouth, to raw forms of fruits with proteins related to the particular allergenic pollens (see the discussion of pollen-associated food allergy syndrome earlier in this chapter). Severe reactions to fruits are less common and are usually not related to pollen allergies. Lipid transfer protein (LTP) syndrome refers to a severe form of allergy to peaches and some other fruits, seeds, and vegetables that share a similar protein, LTP.

What foods are involved with LTP syndrome?

LTP syndrome can result in allergies, possibly severe ones, to multiple foods, including apple, asparagus, barley, cabbage, chestnut, corn, fennel, goji berries, grape, green bean, hazelnut, kiwi, lentil, lettuce, linseed, melon, mustard, orange, peach, peanut, pomegranate, rice, sunflower seed, tomato, walnut, wheat, and others. LTP syndrome is primarily seen in Mediterranean countries and is highly variable regarding which foods are problematic and the severity of reactions among individuals.

Is it possible to be allergic to fruit seeds but not the fruit?

Yes, but this is rare. Reported reactions seem to be related to orange seeds in particular and may be more common in people with severe cashew or pistachio allergies.

Meats

What meats cause allergies?
Allergies to any meats are overall uncommon but can occur with poultry meats (chicken, duck, turkey) and mammalian meats (beef, lamb, pork). Allergies to exotic meats (buffalo, horse, kangaroo, whale, and so on) are also possible.

If I am allergic to chicken, will I be allergic to eggs?
Having a chicken allergy does not usually mean you are at risk for an egg allergy.

If I am allergic to beef, will I be allergic to milk?
Cow's milk allergy is related to beef allergy, as described earlier in this chapter. It is possible to be allergic to beef without having a milk allergy, however.

Is it possible to be allergic to chicken and not turkey?
It is possible, but most people who are allergic to one type are reactive to both.

Does having a poultry allergy mean I will have a mammalian meat allergy (or vice versa)?
No. Poultry allergies are different from mammalian meat allergies.

If I have an allergy to one type of mammalian meat, will I be allergic to others?
Having an allergy to beef likely means having an allergy to veal. Allergy to cow's meat may occur without allergy to other mammals, such as pork or lamb, but there is an increased risk. As in most foods, some proteins in meats are similar to ones in other substances (feather proteins, dog proteins, and so on), but this does not usually translate into other problematic allergies.

Is it possible to have allergic reactions many hours after eating mammalian meats?
There is an uncommon delayed reaction in some people, who develop

typical allergic symptoms (hives, swelling, anaphylaxis) several hours after eating mammalian meats (beef, lamb, pork) or kidneys. People with this problem may also be at risk of reacting to certain cancer treatments that have a similar substance to meat, and to pork- or beef-derived gelatin. The reaction has been traced to allergy to a complex sugar called alpha-gal.

What causes allergy to alpha-gal, and therefore to mammalian meats?

People with delayed allergic reactions to mammalian meats caused by allergy to alpha-gal have typically been bitten by ticks. The tick saliva contains this complex sugar. After time—several years—without tick bites, the allergy may subside.

Fish

What are the different types of fish?

There are many types of fish, including anchovy, bass, catfish, cod, flounder, grouper, haddock, hake, herring, mahi-mahi, perch, pike, pollock, salmon, scrod, snapper, sole, swordfish, tilapia, trout, and tuna. Fish is covered by US labeling laws, which require that the type of fish be named.

If I am allergic to one type of fish and perhaps not others, should I go ahead and eat the ones I can?

Since fish allergy can be severe, you must be vigilant in avoiding triggers. You will need to take special care if you elect to eat some fish when others are a problem (because you may have a mix-up of fish or cross-contact during handling or cooking). This decision should be made in consultation with your allergist, discussing risks and preferences.

I can eat canned fish but not fresh fish. How is this possible?

Canned fish might be tolerated by a person who reacts to less heated forms because the canning process destroys some proteins.

Is it possible to be allergic to all seawater fish but not freshwater fish, or vice versa?

Fish allergy does not usually divide itself in that manner.

What is scombroid fish poisoning?

Spoiled dark-meat scombroid fish (marine fish such as mackerel, sword-fish, tuna) can develop chemicals that are similar to histamine, the chemical released by immune cells during an allergic reaction. Eating the spoiled fish can result in symptoms that mimic an allergic reaction.

Is it possible to be allergic to some parts of a fish and not other parts?

Yes. Fish allergy can be tricky. Allergies to some segments of fish and not others (for example, belly muscle versus side muscle) are not uncommon. For practical purposes, however, avoidance of the entire fish is typically advised.

Where might fish be found as a food or ingredient?

Fish can be an ingredient in unexpected places: Worcestershire sauce and Caesar salad and dressing usually contain fish (anchovies). Caponata, a Sicilian eggplant relish, also may contain anchovies. Surimi, an artificial crabmeat (also known as "sea legs" or "sea sticks"), is made from fish. Fish proteins survive high heat, so if fish is made in a fryer, that fry oil can contaminate otherwise safe foods. Seafood restaurants certainly pose a high risk in general. Ethnic restaurants (such as Chinese, Indonesian, Thai, and Vietnamese) also use fish and fish ingredients in many dishes.

Is fish found in nonfood items?

Fish may be found in cosmetics, medicines, nutritional supplements (for example, omega-3 fatty acids), and pet foods.

If I have a fish allergy, can I use fish oil supplements?

Whether a worrisome amount of fish protein remains in omega-3 fatty acid supplements is unfortunately unclear (but the amount is probably exceedingly low). A discussion with your doctor about the risks is warranted, but alternatives (such as flax oil) are also available.

Can I eat carrageen if I have a fish allergy?

Carrageen is a marine algae, not a fish, and should be safe.

What is anisakis allergy, and how is it related to fish?

Anisakis is a parasite (worm) that can inhabit fish such as herring, mackerel, and sardines and trigger an allergic reaction in someone who eats that fish, which would masquerade as an allergy to that fish. This problem is typically limited to countries where fish is eaten undercooked and never previously frozen.

Does having a fish allergy mean that I would be allergic to caviar?
No. However, some people are allergic to caviar.

Can I eat fish gelatin if I have a fish allergy?
No comprehensive studies have been done to determine whether relevant amounts of fish protein remain in fish-derived gelatin (kosher gelatin). If any proteins remain, the amounts are likely extremely low. Discuss with your allergist whether to avoid this gelatin.

Shellfish

What are the different types of shellfish?
Crustacean shellfish include crab, crawfish, crayfish, crevette, écrevisse, langoustine, lobster, prawn, and shrimp. The non-crustacean types and other sea creatures include abalone, clam, cockle, mussel, octopus, oyster, scallop, snail (escargot), and squid (calamari).

What foods or types of foods might have shellfish proteins?
Shellfish protein may be present in bouillabaisse, fish stock, seafood flavoring (such as crab or clam extract), and surimi. Fish and seafood restaurants are high risk, of course, even when nonshellfish menu items are ordered, because of cross-contact issues during processing and cooking.

Can I get radiocontrast dye if I have a shellfish allergy?
Yes. There is a myth that since there is iodide in radiocontrast dyes used for medical radiographic scans, like computerized tomography (CT) scans, and iodide in shellfish, there is an allergic relationship. This myth stems in part from the misunderstanding that people develop food allergies to iodide, which isn't true. We eat iodide every day in salt. There are no shellfish proteins in radiocontrast dye. The most common reason people have allergic reactions to the dye is because the dye has a high salt concentration, which in some people triggers their allergy cells to release histamine. Although

having a seafood allergy is not directly linked to radiocontrast dye allergy, it is true that people with allergies in general, including food allergies, may be at higher risk of also reacting to radiocontrast dye. Talk to your allergist. Usually, a formulation with a lower concentration of salts is available, or those with a radiocontrast allergy can be premedicated to reduce risks.

Can I take glucosamine chondroitin supplements if I have a shellfish allergy?

Glucosamine chondroitin is an over-the-counter dietary supplement that is derived from shrimp shell and shark cartilage. Presumably, the muscle proteins (which hold the allergens) would not contaminate the product, but this is currently uncertain. Talk to your doctor before trying these supplements.

Do people with shellfish allergy need to avoid chitosan and other chitin products?

Chitosan is derived from the chitin in the shells of shellfish. It is used in bandages, to help blood clot, in dietary supplements with various potential health claims, and in some industrial settings, such as for water filtration and pesticide use. One study evaluating 10 people with shellfish allergy found no response to allergy skin testing with chitosan powder or bandages and no detectable shellfish proteins in the powder. Unfortunately, there is not much information on potential shellfish protein contamination of chitosan, but there is also no reported allergy despite widespread use. Thus, although some caution is warranted, the risk appears to be very low.

If I have a seafood allergy, can I take potassium iodide if there is a radiation emergency?

Yes. People might be given potassium iodide to protect their thyroid in the event of a nuclear emergency. Having a seafood allergy has nothing to do with an iodide allergy, so this treatment should be safe. Allergic reactions to iodide can occur, but these are not like anaphylaxis. Some people develop rashes from iodide-containing medical treatments (such as skin cleansers).

Spices

What foods are spices?

Spices and other seasonings are derived from various plant materials, such as beans, fruit bodies, leaves, roots, seeds, or other plant parts. In general, spice allergies are uncommon, but when they occur, they are similar to those described for fruit, nut, and seed allergies, including the relationship to pollens. Among the spices, mustard is one of the more common allergens.

Is it possible to be allergic to multiple spices?

Yes. Some "spices" are actually combinations of more than one spice; for example, curry may have cumin, pepper, turmeric, and so forth.

How common are allergies to spices?

In general, they are uncommon, but they can be severe. When a person has an allergic reaction to a food and the triggering substance is unclear, I am always interested in determining the exact ingredients, including spices.

Some spices make my nose run. Is that an allergy?

Some spices are spicy because they contain a chemical called capsaicin, which causes the "heat" in foods and may also trigger allergy-like symptoms, including redness and a runny nose. These are chemical and neurologic responses, not an allergic reaction.

Alcoholic Beverages

Is it possible to be allergic to or have allergic-like reactions to wine and spirits?

Yes, in several ways.

Sometimes wine has chemicals, like histamine, that may induce flushing and allergic symptoms. The sulfites in some wines, which are used as preservatives, cause symptoms in people who are sensitive to them, especially asthma symptoms. Some processing agents, such as egg used for clarification, might contribute allergens, but whether these are present in relevant amounts is unclear. Finally, wines and spirits can have allergens from the source ingredients (such as fruits, grains, and nuts).

What food proteins are in alcoholic beverages?
The relevance of residual food proteins in alcoholic beverages has not been extensively studied. As the beverage is made, some proteins may be altered in a way that reduces their allergenicity, but this possibility should not be relied on. Alcoholic beverages are derived from natural ingredients, so fruits, grains, nuts, spices, and other allergenic foods can be components of the beverage. Amaretto is derived from almonds, Frangelico from hazelnuts, and Irish cream from milk. Allergic reactions to beer are uncommon but appear to be related to residual grain proteins.

Miscellaneous Food Allergens and Colors, Additives, Preservatives, and Latex

Babies are supposed to avoid honey. Is this a common allergen?
No. Although it is possible to be allergic to honey, the problem is rare. Babies are not supposed to ingest honey for a different reason. Bacteria in the honey could cause botulism, a type of neurologic problem, if ingested by children under a year of age.

Can people with insect sting allergies eat honey?
Yes.

What is a gelatin allergy?
Gelatin is derived from the skin and bone of beef, pork, or fish. It is an uncommon allergen. The way gelatin is processed may affect its potential to trigger a reaction in an allergic person. For example, gelatin in a soft, jiggly dessert may be less allergenic than gelatin in a chewy gummy candy. The ingredient is also used as a stabilizer in some vaccines, for example, the MMR vaccine. Gelatin allergy can be related to alpha-gal allergy described above.

Can a person with a gelatin allergy eat beef or pork?
Usually. This is because the proteins causing the allergic reactions differ.

However, people with delayed allergic reactions to beef or pork may be at slightly higher risk of gelatin allergy.

Can a person with an allergy to beef or pork gelatin eat fish gelatin?
Yes. There does not appear to be cross-reactivity between mammalian-derived gelatin and fish gelatin.

What unusual food or ingredients can a person be allergic to?
There are many! Almost anything eaten has caused an allergy in someone. Caviar (fish egg) allergy can occur in people who tolerate fish. In China, allergies to bird's nest soup, made in part from saliva of a bird, have triggered reactions. Carmine is a red food dye that is derived from (get ready) the dried body of a beetle, and it has also triggered allergic reactions. Allergies to marijuana are also on record.

Do chemical additives and preservatives cause food allergies?
Yes, but much less often than ones derived from foods, and not in the same way, because the immune system does not respond to chemicals in the way it responds to proteins, which trigger typical allergies.

Can metals in foods cause allergic reactions?
Some people who develop itchy rashes when chemicals or metals come into direct contact with the skin may then develop widespread itchy rashes when they eat foods with the same substance (see the discussion of BHA reactions later in this chapter). Nickel is a metal that can trigger skin sensitivity in some people. For example, they will gradually develop itchy rashes around nickel earrings or necklaces. The same individuals might react to eating nickel in their diet with itchy rashes in various places on the body. If you have this reaction, talk to your doctor about a nickel-free diet. It is not easy, and the effectiveness is somewhat controversial, but it involves letting tap water run before drinking, to avoid leached metals; avoiding utensils with nickel in them and metal food containers and dispensers; and avoiding nickel-containing vitamins and medications as well as particular foods, including almonds, bran, buckwheat, cocoa, hazel, leavened breads, all types of legumes, lettuce, licorice, millet, oatmeal, shellfish, and spinach (this list is not comprehensive).

What natural, nonchemical food additives can cause allergic reactions?

Any additives that contain proteins can cause allergic reactions, although these allergies are rare. Examples include annatto, a yellow color derived from a seed, and saffron, from the dried parts of a flower, which is used for color and flavor. Other food additives that contain proteins are carmine dye (discussed above), gelatin, gums from beans (such as tragacanth). Many foods also can be used to add color—beets, carrots, grape skins, paprika, turmeric, and so forth.

What is pectin?

Pectin is a gelling and thickening agent derived from fruits. Allergic reactions have been rarely described and seem to be a higher risk for persons with cashew or pistachio allergies (although most people with those nut allergies tolerate pectin).

What chemical food additives can cause adverse reactions?

Synthetic colors, preservatives, flavor enhancers, and curing agents are associated with some adverse reactions, but typically not allergic reactions.

What is tartrazine?

Tartrazine (yellow 5) is a synthetic color that has been investigated because of concerns that it may trigger hives, allergic reactions, and asthma.

Does tartrazine cause allergic reactions?

There are several reports of persons who developed nonallergic rashes from this colorant, such as occupational skin rashes. Despite many studies, a connection to asthma has not been proven and appears to be extremely rare, as are nasal reactions.

What are other examples of synthetic colors, and are they related to allergy?

Many other synthetic colors (sunset yellow, erythrosine, ponceau 4R, carmoisine, quinoline yellow, patent blue, and others) have not been proven to cause allergic reactions. Some of these chemicals have been associated with illnesses on rare occasions (rashes, blood vessel disorders), but not typical allergic symptoms.

What is MSG?

MSG, or monosodium glutamate, is a flavor enhancer that occurs naturally in many foods and is used as an additive.

Does MSG cause allergic reactions?

The symptoms attributed to this additive, sometimes called "Asian restaurant syndrome," include burning sensations, tingling, headaches, and drowsiness. Numerous well-designed studies have not been able to routinely reproduce these symptoms in persons believed to be affected. Very large doses, more than would be in typical meals, have reproduced some symptoms, but these are not thought to be allergic reactions.

What are parabens and benzoates?

Parabens and benzoates are preservatives that have been implicated in various allergic-type reactions, including anaphylaxis.

Do parabens and benzoates cause allergic reactions?

Studies suggest that these may rarely (in 2% to 3%) contribute to chronic hives. Benzoates have rarely been identified as a trigger of eczema. Anaphylaxis has been rarely reported.

Do BHA, BHT, nitrites, nitrates, sorbates, and aspartame cause allergic reactions?

There are several additives for which there appear to be a few documented cases of allergic-type reactions, but studies usually do not clearly implicate them. These additives include BHA and BHT (preservatives), nitrites and nitrates (curing agents), sorbates and sorbic acid (preservatives), and aspartame (sweetener). A few people have reportedly become sensitive to BHA through occupational exposure, leading to skin rashes that flared when BHA was eaten. The take-home message is that allergic-type reactions to most additives are extremely rare and, if suspected, should be carefully evaluated further. Usually the suspicion will not be verified, thereby avoiding unnecessary restrictions.

What are sulfites?

Sulfites are added to foods as preservatives or antibrowning agents, or for a bleaching effect. Before 1986, sulfites were used more widely and in larger amounts, particularly on fresh foods such as lettuce.

What are symptoms of sulfite sensitivity?
Sulfites can induce asthma in sensitive persons. The asthma response is believed to be a chemical effect, not a typical allergic response. It seems that the more sulfite a food has, the more likely asthma could result from ingesting it.

What foods are high in sulfites?
Higher amounts of sulfites may be found in dried fruits, lemon juice, sauerkraut, wine vinegar, certain gravies, dried potatoes, and maraschino cherries, among other foods. Sulfites are declared on package labels.

Can sulfites cause nonasthmatic allergic reactions?
Despite a few reports of individuals who appear to have typical allergic reactions to sulfites (hives, anaphylaxis), well-designed studies usually do not confirm such reactions.

Are sulfites in medications a problem if I have sulfite sensitivity?
Sulfites are used to preserve some drugs and have been occasionally associated with triggering asthma. Epinephrine used to treat anaphylaxis has sulfites, but in low amounts that have never been reported to cause a problem (so epinephrine should never be withheld from a person sensitive to sulfites).

If I am sensitive to sulfites, can I use sulfa drugs?
Being sensitive to the preservative sulfite does not mean there is an allergy to medications that have sulfa.

What does latex allergy have to do with food allergy?
Latex is derived from tree sap and therefore has natural proteins that are similar to some food proteins. Because many foods have cross-reacting proteins, however, the relationships can be overwhelming to untangle and determine what foods might be allergenic to someone with latex allergy. Some latex-related troublemakers are bananas and kiwis. These two fruits have interrelationships with each other, pollens, and latex. Also related to latex allergy are avocados, bell peppers, chestnuts, figs, mangoes, peaches, potatoes, and tomatoes. These relationships are complex, and most people with an allergy to any one of these foods (or to latex) tolerate the others. If you do not already eat and tolerate the food related to your allergy, however, discuss with your doctor whether to avoid the food.

Case Studies

Was it an allergy?

Case 1. Five-year-old Louie developed hives an hour after eating shrimp six months ago. His family knew shrimp was a common allergen, so they stopped giving it to him and came for an allergy evaluation. I learned that Louie loved a wide variety of foods and had continued to eat lobster and crab over the months following the apparent reaction to shrimp. I knew that it is unusual to be allergic to shrimp and not lobster or crab. Had Louie eaten some other unusual ingredient at the meal? Was there some other potential trigger of hives?

After I asked more questions, I learned that Louie had been ill with a fever for about three days before the "reaction" and that the hives lasted for three days. I explained that hives, although often a sign of allergy, can also develop from infections. It is very unusual for a food to trigger hives lasting more than a few hours, and so I was convinced, given all of the details, that Louie could go back to eating shrimp and no allergy tests were needed. Not an allergy.

Case 2. Forty-year-old Marsha was having dinner with her work colleagues. The dinner included tuna, asparagus, and potatoes. She developed a feeling of itching all over, some throat tightness, and flushing. She went to the emergency room and was treated for an allergic reaction. I learned that Marsha had never had any allergic problems throughout her lifetime. She stopped eating tuna after the incident but ate other fish without a problem. She also ate all of the other ingredients of the meal without incident. I asked her if any of her colleagues also ordered the tuna, but she did not think so. I performed an allergy skin test to tuna, and it was negative. We called the restaurant and found out that two other patrons had experienced a similar illness from the tuna. I diagnosed scombroid fish poisoning and explained how it is a masquerader of food allergy. So this was not an allergy.

Case 3. Sally had experienced several mystery reactions. She had hives and coughing from three meals, but the ingredients of all of the meals were known, and none were problematic. For example, her dinner of fish contained ingredients she usually tolerates. Her lunch with a seasoned rice and salad was typical. And even her beverages—iced tea, lemonade, or coffee—

were her usual. My only clue was that Sally had a severe cashew allergy. She had prior severe reactions with trace exposure to cashew, and her tests to cashew were at the top of the charts. Knowing that some people who are sensitive to cashew also react to citrus seeds, pectin, or pink peppercorn, I asked about the possibility of those ingredients. We determined that reactions to the three meals were likely due to her having cut fresh lemons, leading to inclusion of crushed pieces of lemon seed in the lemonade, on the fish, and in the rice. Yes, this was an allergy.

CHAPTER 2

When and How to Discuss a Possible Food Allergy Diagnosis with Your Doctor

This chapter answers questions about when and how to seek a food allergy diagnosis.

When to Talk to Your Doctor

When should I suspect a food allergy?

If you or your child experience symptoms of allergy, such as hives (like mosquito bites), rashes, swelling, itching, coughing, wheezing, or vomiting soon after eating a food, you should suspect a food allergy. There are also several chronic health problems that could be related to foods.

Why should I see a doctor for my or my child's food allergies?

It is essential to confirm a food allergy so the person with the allergy can avoid the allergenic foods and a treatment plan can be put in place for any severe allergies.

When should I discuss my suspicion of food allergy with my doctor?

As soon as possible. You would not want to avoid a food that is not causing any problems, and you certainly would want to confirm any triggers so that you can remain healthy by avoiding them.

Why not self-diagnose a food allergy?

When a person suspects a food allergy, they are often incorrect about the cause of their symptoms.

What type of doctor should I see if I suspect a food allergy?

You should start with your primary care doctor. They might identify a cause of your symptoms that is not an allergy, or they may give a referral to an allergist-immunologist.

Why see an allergist for food allergies?

An allergist, also called an allergist-immunologist, is a specialist who has received additional training in the diagnosis and management of food allergies and has access to additional tests to confirm or exclude an allergy.

How to Prepare for a Doctor Visit

What should I do before seeing the doctor about a possible food allergy?

To help your doctor make a diagnosis, you should write down all details of the problems you have experienced. It is easy to get overwhelmed at a doctor's visit, and having things written down can be helpful. Record the symptoms, how long you have had them, their timing in relation to any foods, and the details about your diet that may inform your doctor of possible triggers. See table 2.1 for a list of information for your doctor and from your doctor.

What is a diet record?

A diet record shows what you are eating, when, and any symptoms. You can compose a diet record on lined paper. Write down all the ingredients of foods and beverages, what you were doing at the time you experienced symptoms (exercise, resting, etc.), and any medications you were taking. If the symptoms are repetitive or chronic, it is helpful to include meals that you seem to tolerate. You may wish to record several days of typical meals and symptoms. Table 2.2 is an example of a diet record. From this example record, we might become suspicious that raw egg is causing symptoms.

Table 2.1. Things to Consider When Preparing for the Doctor Visit

	General Issues	Details
Things I need to tell the doctor	Symptoms	Timing, relation to meals or specific foods
		Any activities related to the symptoms
	Diet information	Ingredient labels from products causing symptoms, diet diaries
	General medical information	List of medications (bring them)
		Any lab tests, medical records, referral letters, pharmacy information
	What I hope to get from this visit	What is causing problems, what can I eat or should avoid, how to manage the problem, what will happen with time
	Other:	
Things I need to ask the doctor	What can I eat, and what should I not eat?	Ask for specifics about foods and food groups
		Discuss severity
	What do the tests mean?	Discuss all results
	How do I manage the allergy day to day?	Consider restaurants, travel, school, when and how to use medications
	What is the prognosis?	
	Are there treatments?	
	What do I do next? When do I return?	
	Other:	

Table 2.2. Example Diet Record

Date	Meal	Symptoms	Details
Monday 12th	Breakfast: scrambled egg, coffee with milk, strawberries	Lip swelling 5 minutes after eating the meal, stomach pain 10 minutes later	Eggs were runny

Had taken medicine for headache |
| | Lunch: turkey, mustard, wheat bread, sesame on bread, Swiss cheese, chocolate chip cookie, tea | No problems | Cookie ingredient list attached |
| | Dinner: hamburger on a sesame bun, lemon soda, tomato, ketchup, lettuce, potato fries in canola oil, meringue cookies | Lip swelling and throat itch started after the cookies | Ingredient list of homemade meringue cookies attached |

Why should I keep a diet record?

If it is not clear what triggered your symptoms, you and your doctor can review the relationship to specific meals. The allergenic food will usually trigger symptoms each time it is eaten, so the diet record may help to narrow the possibilities. Make sure all the ingredients are listed, especially for meals that triggered symptoms.

Are there ways to narrow down which foods might be causing symptoms?

Remember that foods eaten often without symptoms are not as likely to be triggers as the accidental inclusion of a known allergen (a nut, for example, when you already know you have tree nut allergies) or a new allergy to an ingredient that you do not commonly ingest (for example, some spice that you do not eat often).

Are there circumstances around the time of a meal that could cause me to have a reaction to a food I usually tolerate?

Absolutely. If you have a reaction that seems to be to a food you usually tolerate, you should think about different variables. Did you eat more of something than usual? Were you taking any medications, including over-the-counter ones? Did you exercise after the meal? Did you have alcohol with the meal? Were you ill, with fever? Were you menstruating? These additional circumstances sometimes enhance the response to a potential food allergen.

What is the value of bringing ingredient labels to a doctor visit?

Sometimes a minor or hidden ingredient is the cause of a reaction. Having the ingredient label on hand may help to identify an otherwise unsuspected trigger.

How do I obtain ingredient information from manufacturers?

Most ingredients will be listed on a label. But vague terms are sometimes used to hide proprietary ingredients. For example, terms such as "spices" or "flavors" may be used. You can contact a manufacturer to try to get those "secret ingredients," but it may be difficult. You may wish to ask your doctor about the possibility of a hidden ingredient being the trigger, and then work together to obtain more information from the manufacturer if needed.

How do I obtain ingredient information from a restaurant?

Discuss the ingredients in a nonaccusatory manner. Explain that you are concerned about a food allergy and want to consider any possible ingredients. If you have a known allergy and experience a reaction at a restaurant, promptly inform the restaurant and discuss the preparation to determine whether the reaction could have been to accidental inclusion of your known trigger(s) or to another ingredient that may be a new problem.

Would I need to be off any medications prior to the office visit?

For your first visit with your primary care doctor, you likely do not need to avoid any medications. An allergist may request that you avoid antihistamines and some other medications that may block results to allergy skin testing. Asthma medications and most other medications can be continued. Table 2.3 describes some medications that interfere with allergy skin tests. These do not interfere with allergy blood tests.

Table 2.3. Examples of Common Medications That Interfere with Allergy Skin Testing

Type	Specific Medications	Days to Be Off
Antihistamines	Brompheniramine, chlorpheniramine, diphenhydramine	Stop 1–3 days before
	Azelastine, cetirizine, fexofenadine, hydroxyzine, loratadine	Stop 3–10 days before
Antidepressants, tranquilizers, and appetite stimulants	Doxepin, imipramine, periactin, phenothiazines	Ask your doctor; can last days to weeks

Note: Talk to your doctor before stopping any medication. Stopping a medication could cause illness. Asthma medications do not have to be stopped. Watch for ingredients in eye drops and nasal sprays. The following common allergy medications do not affect skin tests: short-term oral or topical use of steroids, cromolyn, asthma inhalers, montelukast, or acid blockers like ranitidine and cimetidine.

Should I bring suspect foods with me to the doctor visit?

Especially if you are seeing an allergist, you may want to bring any unusual ingredients (such as spices, seeds, or exotic fruits) that were in the meal that triggered a reaction or that you suspect may be an allergen. The allergist may use that food to perform a skin test.

If I had a reaction to a packaged food or restaurant meal, should I bring that to the visit?

If it is not clear what triggered the reaction, it may be helpful to bring the actual foods, along with any ingredient lists or labels. Wrap the foods and label them "DO NOT EAT," then freeze them until the allergy visit.

What will the doctor do during the visit to evaluate for food allergy?

The doctor should take a careful medical history, perform a physical examination, and consider any testing, if needed.

What is the doctor looking for in the medical history?

The medical history is crucial for the physician to consider whether food allergy is the correct diagnosis or to determine an alternative one. The doctor will consider whether the symptoms are typical of allergy or related to specific foods, or the doctor might have alternative explanations. All these clues are in the discussion you have with the doctor and any records you may have.

What is the doctor looking for during the physical examination?
Sometimes there are rashes or other physical evidence of allergy or of illnesses that may provide an alternative explanation for the symptoms.

What tests might the doctor perform?
A primary care doctor may perform a blood test. An allergist may perform blood tests as well as allergy skin tests and other tests. These tests and others are explained in detail in chapter 3.

Finding the Right Doctor and Other Health Professionals

How do I find a doctor who cares for people with food allergy?
A board-certified allergist-immunologist is specifically trained to diagnose and treat food allergies. You may discuss a referral with your primary care doctor. You can also search for doctors near you by zip code on www.aaaai .org, the website for the American Academy of Allergy, Asthma, and Immunology, or on www.acaai.org, the website for the American College of Allergy, Asthma, and Immunology. The lay organization Food Allergy Research & Education (FARE) has compiled a "Clinical Network" of 50 institutions that collaborate to advance the field of food allergy and promote clinical care (https://www.foodallergy.org/research-innovation/elevating-research /fare-clinical-network).

What qualifications should I look for in an allergist to treat my food allergies?
As you would want from any doctor, the allergist should be compassionate, ready to listen carefully to your concerns, and willing to explain diagnosis and treatment to your satisfaction. Friends or relatives may have advice on a good doctor. I recommend seeing an allergist who is certified by the American Board of Allergy and Immunology (or a similar certifying board outside the United States).

What is a board-certified allergist-immunologist?

This certification is given to a physician who was initially trained and certified to be a pediatrician, internist, or both, and has completed an additional two to three years of training in a fellowship learning the care of allergic disorders, including asthma, hay fever, anaphylaxis, food allergy, insect sting allergy, and immune system problems. Certification requires passing a final test, and maintaining the certification requires ongoing educational activities and periodic retesting.

How do I determine whether my allergist is board certified?

You can check on the website of the American Board of Allergy and Immunology at www.abai.org.

What other health professionals care for food allergy?

A gastroenterologist may be helpful in the care of chronic gut symptoms related to food allergies. A registered dietitian may be helpful in treatment.

Why would I see a dietitian?

When foods are removed from the diet because of allergies, there could be nutritional deficits. A registered dietitian can evaluate the diet to ensure that proper substitutes or supplements are providing appropriate nutrition. The dietitian can also provide advice regarding food allergen avoidance.

What is the difference between a dietitian, a nutritionist, and a dietetic technician?

They have different training and expertise. Whatever specialist you choose, it can be helpful to discuss their experience with food allergies. If your child is the patient, confirm the practitioner's experience with pediatric concerns.

What is a registered dietitian?

A registered dietitian (RD) has earned a bachelor's degree, completed an accredited practice program, passed a qualifying examination, and is required to continue educational activities to maintain certification. The degree indicates expertise in food and nutrition. Some registered dietitians may also refer to themselves as nutritionists.

What is a nutritionist?

A person with the title of nutritionist may have forms of training that differ from those of a registered dietitian, with varying types of certification based on the state in which the nutritionist practices.

What is a registered dietetic technician?

A registered dietetic technician has earned a two-year associate's degree and completed 450 hours of supervised practice (about half the hours of a registered dietitian).

Complementary and Alternative Therapies

What about seeing a naturalist, alternative medicine practitioner, or acupuncturist?

Several nontraditional practitioners address food allergies. Alternative medicine typically implies using only non-mainstream approaches. Complementary medicine refers to using non-mainstream approaches in addition to mainstream ones. Many people pursue evaluation and treatment from nontraditional practitioners. Treatments may include probiotics, herbs, acupuncture, and other approaches. Many people report results, but there is limited careful scientific study. Regarding food allergies, studies are underway. Exploring these alternatives is a buyer-beware situation, and it is advisable to pursue traditional medical evaluations and treatments as well. Unproven and disproven methods are reviewed in chapter 3.

Are there any dangers to alternative therapies for food allergy?

I do not have a strong feeling against people trying alternative means. I also understand people wanting to investigate treatment options, but I do worry about problems that could arise. For example, abandoning routine treatment could lead to a bad outcome while emphasis is directed toward another therapy that is unproven. Practitioners of many alternative therapies are not monitored. Unproven treatments, even when they are "natural," could have side effects. In fact, there is an apparent misconception that alternative therapies are automatically safer than standard Western pharmaceutical approaches. It should be appreciated that many medications we routinely use today were initially derived from plants. They differ from alternative remedies primarily in that standard medications are typically well studied, side effects are known, and manufacturing is standardized.

Herbal products in the United States are not regulated, ingredients can vary, and the products can remain on shelves as long as they are not proven to be unsafe. Nonetheless, it is possible to have side effects from herbal treatments, including allergic reactions. Overall, natural remedies are a constant buyer-beware situation.

CHAPTER 3

All about Allergy Tests

This chapter answers questions about allergy tests: How are they selected and interpreted? How do skin tests compare with blood tests? What are the newest tests? And many others.

General Questions about Testing

What is the most important test to diagnose a food allergy?
The medical history. Although not often thought of as a "test," a person's medical history is much more important than any blood or skin tests for allergy.

Why is the medical history so important for diagnosing a food allergy?
As described in chapter 2, your doctor needs to know details about symptoms and diet to determine whether food allergy is a possibility, as well as to decide if additional tests are needed and which tests to perform. The tests are only helpful when they are interpreted in the context of your medical history.

Can a food allergy be diagnosed by medical history alone?
Sometimes the medical history makes a diagnosis obvious. For example, if a person repeatedly develops severe allergy symptoms minutes after eating a particular food, a diagnosis of allergy to that food is evident. Nonetheless, experts recommend a confirmatory test.

What tests are used to diagnose a food allergy?
Allergy skin tests and blood tests are most often used. These tests detect IgE antibodies, the immune system protein that causes many types of

allergic reactions to foods, as described in chapter 1. Additional tests are elimination diets and feeding tests.

How are allergy tests used to diagnose a food allergy?

Skin and blood tests are selected and interpreted in the context of the medical history to provide additional evidence for or against an allergy to a specific food. Feeding tests (the medical term is oral food challenge) give the most definitive evidence about a food allergy.

What foods can be tested?

Essentially any foods can be tested. Companies make extracts for skin testing and blood tests for many foods. Not all foods have commercial tests, however. As described below, an allergist may be able to create a test using the food itself.

Are there tests for dyes, preservatives, and food colors?

Although tests can be made for these substances, reactions to them, as described in chapter 2, are generally not caused by IgE unless the trigger has proteins (that is, an additive derived from a natural substance, like a seed).

Skin Tests

What are allergy skin tests?

An allergy skin test is a quick and simple way to determine whether the body has made IgE antibodies to the food being tested.

How are allergy skin tests performed?

A small amount of liquid extract of the food being tested is introduced into the top layer of skin using a metal or plastic probe to scratch the skin surface. Because the skin is scratched, or "pricked," these tests are often called scratch tests or skin prick tests. In addition to the foods being tested, saltwater and histamine tests are placed with the probe.

Where are the skin tests placed?

The tests are placed on a rash-free area of the less hairy part of the forearm or back.

What foods can be tested by skin tests?

Commercial extracts of more than a hundred foods are approved for testing. An allergist can also make tests from whole fresh foods.

Why are fresh raw or whole foods sometimes used for allergy skin tests?

Commercially prepared extracts are most often used to test for food allergies. Sometimes an unusual food (such as beans, exotic fruit, specific fish, seeds, or spices) without a commercial extract must be tested, so allergists make their own extracts. Sometimes the commercial extract is missing some proteins that were lost in processing or storage, and the doctor may elect to use a fresh extract to avoid missing a diagnosis if the medical history indicates a possible allergy. This is sometimes called prick-prick testing, as the allergist pricks the food and then the person being tested.

What does a positive test look like?

Like a mosquito bite. There is a raised center and surrounding redness. When positive, the raised center usually has a width measurement that is between the size of a pea and a nickel.

Why is a histamine skin test performed while doing food skin tests?

Histamine is a chemical released from allergy cells that causes symptoms such as itching, swelling, and redness. The histamine skin test result should be positive, showing that the tests were reliable and not suppressed by any medications. The test represents an average positive for comparison. The histamine in the test is manufactured; it is not from people.

Why is a saltwater skin test performed while doing food skin tests?

Salt water produces a negative result for comparison. No one is allergic to salt water (saline), but some people develop swelling just from the skin irritation of being scratched. This test allows the doctor to take this nonspecific irritation response into account when evaluating the food tests.

What are the food allergy skin tests measuring?

IgE antibodies to the food that was tested. A positive test occurs when a person's immune system has made IgE antibodies that recognize the proteins in the test. If this is the case, doctors say that the person is "sensitized" to the tested food.

At what age can skin tests be performed?
Any age. Even infants can be tested.

Are the food allergy skin tests accurate in infants and young children?
They are helpful at any age; however, infants are slightly more likely to register a negative test despite having an allergy.

Do the skin tests hurt?
No. Most people feel a slight discomfort during the scratch, similar to a fingernail scratching the skin. There is no bleeding. The positive tests become itchy, but this is usually mild and goes away quickly.

Is there anything I can do to make the tests less uncomfortable?
Most infants do not cry because the discomfort is minimal. Children may be more likely to cry out of fright, so addressing their fear of the test is helpful. Distracting a child with a song, video, story, or other means may lessen the anxiety. After the doctor reads the results, a cool compress may be soothing, but this is often not necessary. If there is significant itching, an antihistamine can be taken or a cream applied.

How long until a result is obtained from the skin test?
Positive tests may begin to show in minutes. The doctor will read the results 10 to 20 minutes after the test is performed.

What should I do while the tests are developing?
Don't scratch! Rubbing the test could affect the results. Children may be kept busy with a game or other distraction. It is okay to roll down sleeves or put a shirt back on to cover the test areas as they are developing.

How does the doctor record the skin test result?
The size of the bump in the middle of the response is measured. Doctors may record the size in various ways, and they may also measure the redness surrounding the bump. The bump is called a wheal, and the redness is called the flare.

How long before the skin test bumps go away?
The itching usually subsides in about 10 to 20 minutes, and the bumps generally fade within an hour, although sometimes they last much longer, depending on their size.

Can the skin test bumps come back?

Rarely, a bump reappears a few hours later only to fade again.

Can skin tests cause allergic reactions?

When positive, the test causes a small, local allergic reaction on the skin surface just where the scratch was made. Since allergens are being scratched into the skin, there is a very small risk of an allergic reaction beyond the spot that was pricked.

What is the risk of a severe reaction from skin testing?

Allergic reactions such as nasal symptoms or spreading hives or a more severe reaction happen in fewer than 1 in 1,000 people being tested and are usually associated with having large numbers of tests at once, with many of them registering positive.

Are there situations when skin tests cannot be done?

Sometimes, if a person has extensive rashes, there is nowhere to put the test.

Are there situations when skin tests should not be done?

If antihistamines have been used recently, the tests can be blocked, and testing should be postponed.

Is it okay to do a skin test to a food that caused severe anaphylaxis?

If there is a recent history of severe anaphylaxis and one specific food was clearly the cause, many allergists will opt to use a blood test rather than a skin test for confirmation because the skin test will likely be positive, and the reaction may be larger and more uncomfortable. However, it would not be wrong to go forward with a skin test to obtain quick confirmation of the allergy.

Can skin tests cause a food allergy?

Experts do not think so. No comprehensive studies confirm this conclusion, but many factors suggest this is not a concern.

Do I need to stop taking any medications to prepare for having skin tests?

Yes, you need to stop taking medications that block the skin test results. See table 2.3 in chapter 2.

Is there a way for the allergist to check if I have been off antihistamines long enough to be tested?
Yes. If you are not sure, the allergist can begin by placing just a histamine test. If this test causes a sufficiently large response, the remainder of the planned tests can be placed. Otherwise, testing would be postponed.

What do I do if I need an avoided medication before an appointment for skin testing?
Take it. Your allergist may be able to perform blood tests instead because antihistamines do not affect blood tests, or you can reschedule the skin tests. A single dose may not interrupt the tests, so call ahead and explain what you took and when.

How many skin tests should be done?
There is no exact answer to this question because tests should be selected based on suspicions about which foods might be causing symptoms. Usually only a few foods are being considered as potential triggers at any one time, so selection of relevant foods is unlikely to require more than 10 to 15 tests.

Should I be tested to every food to see what I might be allergic to?
There is certainly no reason to test any foods already in the diet that are not causing any symptoms. Also, the tests have limited accuracy, so they do not give definitive "yes or no" results. For these and other reasons, your doctor should select foods that make sense as potential allergens warranting a test.

What does a positive or negative skin test mean?
A positive test means that the body has made IgE antibodies that recognize the protein in the test. This is called being sensitized. A negative test means that no such IgE has been detected.

Is a person ever able to eat the food anyway after a positive skin test?
Yes, yes, and YES!

Why can some people eat the food anyway despite a positive skin test?
The skin test detects that the immune system has made IgE antibodies to a food, but having IgE antibodies to a food often happens in people who are nonetheless able to eat the food. This is why the medical history is so crucial for proper test selection and interpretation.

Can a skin test be negative and a person still be allergic?

Yes, but not often.

Why would a skin test be negative in a person who is actually allergic?

Four reasons. First, although uncommon, the extract may be lacking a protein to which a person is allergic. Foods are made of many different proteins, and some of them may be underrepresented in a test. If a person is allergic to a protein from the food that is missing in the test extract, the test will be falsely negative. In this case, if suspicion is high, another test could be performed, such as a skin test with fresh, raw food or a blood test. Second, the person may have a type of allergy that is not caused by IgE antibodies, so the test result is not relevant. Third, the use of antihistamines may have blocked the result, although this would likely have also blocked the histamine comparison test. And fourth, there could have been human error, in which case the test can be repeated.

Why would a test be positive if the person can eat the food?

One explanation has to do with digestion. When the food is placed on the skin for testing, it is not digested. There may be IgE antibodies that recognize the undigested protein, leading to the skin response—a positive test. After the food is eaten, the proteins become digested and may not be recognized by those same IgE antibodies. Therefore the skin test is positive, but the food is tolerated when eaten. Another explanation has to do with the amount of IgE antibodies. There may be enough to cause a skin response or be detected in a blood test but not enough to activate enough allergy cells to cause symptoms when the food is eaten.

Are the skin tests accurate?

Yes. They are excellent for detecting IgE antibodies to the protein being tested. But they must be interpreted in the context of the medical history because a positive test alone does not prove a true allergy.

What would be an example of using a test result and a history together to diagnose a food allergy?

Let's suppose you had an itchy mouth during a meal in which sesame and mustard were the only foods you did not routinely eat. If the sesame test was positive and the mustard test was negative, then the evidence is strongest that the sesame was the culprit. But if you were tested to wheat, which was also in the meal, and it was positive, that would not diagnose a wheat allergy, because you eat wheat all the time without a problem. That wheat test should not even have been performed.

Why are the skin test bumps measured or "graded" in size?
The larger the bump, or wheal, the more likely the food tested is truly a problem.

Do skin tests predict the severity of an allergy?
No.

Why would skin wheal size not reflect the severity of an allergy?
The larger the wheal, the more likely that the food tested is a problem. Multiple factors influence severity, however. The allergy test does not know if you have asthma (associated with more severe reactions), how much of the food you might have eaten (the more eaten, the worse a reaction might be), or your state of health at the time of an allergic reaction. This is why wheal size is not a good predictor of an allergy's severity.

Blood Tests (and How They Compare with Skin Tests)

What blood tests are available for food allergy testing?
There are commercial blood tests for allergy to well over a hundred different foods.

What are the food allergy blood tests measuring?
IgE antibodies that the immune system has made against the proteins of foods in the test.

Why does a doctor perform a blood test for food allergy?
To determine whether, and how much, food-specific IgE antibodies are in the bloodstream.

What does a positive or negative blood test mean?
A positive test indicates the presence of IgE antibodies to the tested food, and a negative test indicates that the test did not detect these antibodies.

How are blood test results reported?

The test might be reported as classes, counts, or units. The different methods of reporting have to do with tradition and technical aspects of the test. Nowadays, an increasing number of laboratories are reporting the results in units called kIU/L or kU_A/L.

What does kIU/L or kU_A/L mean?

It stands for a measure of units per liter. This is similar to a concentration, such as how much of something is in a specified space. In this case, it is the amount of IgE that is specific to the food allergen. In this format, the test runs from "undetectable," usually signified by <0.1 or sometimes <0.35, to a high of >100. The < symbol means "less than," and the > symbol means "greater than."

Can blood test results from different laboratories be compared?

It depends. If laboratories are using the same approved, automated test system for all your tests, the results can be compared. But currently there are three test systems in use. Each of the three manufacturers creates its food test in a slightly different way, so results from one system's manufacturer may not be exactly the same as those from another. Your doctor should know which test system the laboratories are using.

Can a blood test be positive and not indicate a food allergy?

Yes. The test accurately measures IgE antibodies to the food, but a person can have IgE antibodies to a food and tolerate eating the food anyway.

If a blood test is negative, can there still be a food allergy?

Yes. This can occur because either the type of allergy being evaluated does not depend on IgE antibodies, or the proteins from the food in the test did not include ones that are relevant to the particular individual. Rarely, there can be a laboratory error as well. When results do not make sense, the test might be repeated, or another test, such as the skin test, might be performed.

What is an example of when a blood test was negative but there was an allergy anyway?

A patient who had a severe reaction to bananas had negative skin and blood tests to bananas. She clearly had symptoms that were severe when she was

Complete Guide to Food Allergies

eating a banana, however, and no other foods or explanations made sense. When she was skin tested using a bit of raw banana, the test was positive. This confirmed her allergy and suggested that the previous tests had been negative because she was sensitive to a protein present primarily in the raw preparation. The extracts and blood test missed that protein for this patient.

What does a higher blood test result mean?
The higher the result, the stronger the positive test and the more likely a true food allergy is present. The case is the same for skin tests—the larger the wheal/bump, the more likely there is a true allergy. Figure 3.1 illustrates how allergy tests (reflecting chance of allergy) differ from yes-no tests, like those for pregnancy.

Can a blood test for allergy be so strongly positive that it confirms a definite allergy?
In some circumstances, yes. Studies in children using the ImmunoCAP test have shown that almost all children with particularly high test results had true allergies. Table 3.1 summarizes some of the studies. These numbers are only a rough guide. There are only a few studies relating allergy outcomes to the test results, and the results differ, so the numbers may not always apply. Most foods have not been adequately studied, nor have the various manufacturers' tests. Therefore it is important for allergists to interpret each test in light of individual circumstances.

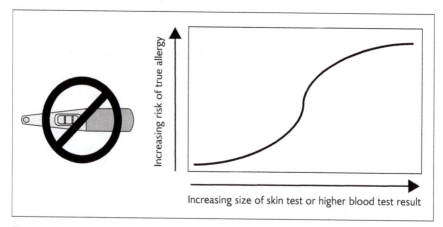

Figure 3.1. Food allergy skin and blood tests are not like a pregnancy test; they do not give a yes-or-no result. Instead, they are a statistic that reflects the chance of allergy.

Table 3.1. Examples of Blood Test Results above Which a True Allergy Is Very Likely, but Not Certain

Food	Value at or above Which Allergy Is Very Likely (kU$_A$/L)
Cow's milk (whole forms)	15
Egg (like scrambled egg)	7
Fish	20
Peanut	15
Sesame	50
Tree nuts	20

Note: Circumstances of age, history, other allergies, underlying illnesses, and other factors affect the results.

How does the relationship between a test result and a food vary by age?
Based on limited studies, specific values seem related to higher risk for younger children. For example, a test result of 2 kU$_A$/L for a 1-year-old may be high and associated with a strong risk of allergy, while the same result may be unlikely to indicate an allergy in a 10-year-old. The relationship has not been studied in adults.

Is there a low positive blood test result that guarantees there is no allergy to the food?
Although lower test results are more favorable indicators that a food will be tolerated, no results by themselves are definitive to exclude an allergy. But if the medical history is not compelling and the test is negative, the food can usually be excluded as a trigger.

How are the blood tests different from the skin tests?
The tests are more similar than different. They both measure IgE antibodies to the food being tested.

Which is more accurate, skin or blood tests?
Both tests are excellent at detecting even small amounts of food-specific IgE antibodies. Sometimes one test will be positive while the other is negative.

Why does the accuracy differ among tests?

The tests are made by extracting proteins from the foods. Each food is a collection of many different proteins, and an individual with an allergy may be reacting to any of them. Different manufacturers of skin test extracts and of the blood tests use different techniques to extract the proteins. There may be subtle differences in the amount and types of proteins from one particular food that each test can measure. Therefore the test results differ sometimes, favoring either a skin or a blood test.

How does a doctor decide whether to do the skin test, the blood test, or both?

Both tests give similar information, but a doctor selects one, the other, or both based on medical circumstances. Often, the skin test is performed when an immediate result is desired or an unexpected result occurred from a blood test. The blood test is often used to monitor an allergy over time, because it is easier to compare results from one year to the next with a blood test than it is with a skin test.

What is an example of why you might pick one test in particular?

Let's consider a child who, according to her mother, had a rash flare when eating eggs on two separate occasions. I assume that the child does have an egg allergy because the story is consistent, and I am interested in monitoring the allergy over time. I send a blood test to the lab, and it comes back showing an undetectable level, $<0.1 \, kU_A/L$. This is a surprise, so I have the family return. The mother now wonders if maybe something else was in the food, for example, cinnamon. I perform a skin test for egg and for cinnamon, and only the egg test is positive. This is an example where the skin test was a bit more sensitive than the blood test, and indeed it was an egg allergy all along.

Do I need to avoid any medications before having the blood tests?

No.

How many foods can be tested in the blood test?

It is conceivable to order many dozens of tests, but this is usually not necessary. Tests should be selected on the basis of one's medical history, and usually this means testing fewer than a dozen foods. The number of foods that could be tested is limited only by the amount of blood taken.

What are food allergy "panel" tests?

To make testing convenient, manufacturers create panels of tests so that a doctor can check a box and obtain groups of tests, rather than indicating each food separately. These panels might be for common food allergens, such as eggs, milk, peanuts, wheat, and soy. Or they might represent groups of foods, such as tree nuts.

Should I be tested to a panel of "everything"?

No. Because tests are not able to diagnose an allergy by themselves, it is not a good idea to indiscriminately have dozens or even hundreds of tests performed. Many tests will be positive for foods that are actually completely innocent and tolerated components in the diet, and these positives can be misleading.

Should I be tested to a panel of foods that are related to one that caused an allergy?

It depends. Considering your medical history and understanding the relationships of foods are the first steps. For a person allergic to peanuts, which are a type of bean, positive test results for other beans, such as soy, pea, and string bean, are common (over 50%), but true allergy to the other beans occurs in only about 5% to 20% of people with peanut allergies, depending upon the bean being considered. In this situation, testing to a panel of beans could give misleading positive results. Test selection must be based in part on what the person is already eating and tolerating and what the person may not have eaten and may be at risk for, among other factors.

Why would a doctor decide to test me to a panel of foods?

Unfortunately, doctors sometimes inappropriately use test panels for convenience. Rather than individually picking the needed tests, they might just send a preselected "panel" to save time. Although this approach is not unreasonable, it can create confusion and anxiety when results are positive to foods that are otherwise of no concern. In some cases, however, panels of tests are appropriate to screen for possible allergy. An example would be a young child who reacted to a single tree nut but has not tried to ingest any other tree nuts. In this case, an allergist might order a panel of tests to tree nuts to determine which among the group could pose a risk.

Why would a doctor decide not to test me to a panel of foods?

There is really no reason to test for a food that is already tolerated in the diet and for which there is no concern of allergy. For example, testing a panel that includes milk, egg, soy, and wheat is not necessary for a person already eating those foods without any symptoms or chronic illnesses that raise suspicions of allergy to those foods.

Does the blood test predict the severity of an allergy?

No. At least not very well. A few studies suggest that people with a higher test result might be more prone to severe reactions, but other studies do not show this pattern.

Why wouldn't a blood test reflect severity of an allergy?

The higher the test result, the more likely the food poses a problem. Different factors relate to severity. The allergy test does not know if you have asthma, how much of the food you might have eaten, or your state of health at the time of an allergic reaction. The test does not know how your cells might react. The standard tests are evaluating the immune response to a selection of proteins in the food, and some of those proteins are more potent than others in some foods. Therefore the standard tests may not reflect allergic responses to allergens within a food that causes more severe reactions.

What are the advantages of a blood test over a skin test?

The blood test is not affected by your taking antihistamines, does not require rash-free areas of skin for testing, and can easily be compared from time to time, so long as the same manufacturer is used.

What are the advantages of a skin test over a blood test?

The skin test gives an immediate result, can be performed with fresh or whole foods if necessary, and is much less costly than the blood test.

If the tests are not perfect, why are they done at all?

They help to provide additional evidence for or against an allergy.

Does having had a recent allergic reaction affect the test results?

There is a theoretical concern that having had a recent severe reaction might "use up" a lot of the IgE antibodies being tested, resulting in a lower or a negative test result. In practicality, we do not usually see this, but an allergist would retest in a few weeks if the test results were suspiciously negative after a severe reaction.

Can both the skin test and blood tests be negative even when there is an allergy?

Yes. This can happen if the illness is not associated with having IgE antibodies to the food (non-IgE-mediated, or cell-mediated, reactions as described in chapter 1) or because the tests did not have the right proteins.

Can you give an example of how the tests might not have the right proteins?

Sesame allergy is an example. Some of the proteins that cause allergic reactions to sesame are oil based. The skin and blood tests, however, are made from the water-based proteins. It is difficult to make tests from oil-based proteins. Therefore, if a person has a convincing allergic reaction to sesame but the tests are negative, I remain suspicious and may try to test with the oil from sesame.

If the blood test results rise or fall over time, what does that mean?

Test results going down with time may indicate that an allergy is resolving. Results going up may indicate that the allergy is persisting. Sometimes, the test stays the same even though the person is resolving the allergy. Because high or low results reflect the chance of a true allergy, not the severity, what the result is at any point in time is as important as whether it is getting stronger or weaker.

Why do allergy test results go up or down when the food is not being eaten?

We do not know why test results rise, fall, or stay the same. When a test shows increase, it usually means the allergy is not waning. Whether the food was eaten does not appear to relate to this rise. One explanation could be that the body's total production of IgE is increasing, so the antibodies to the food being tested are simply rising along with it (similar to a child growing). Perhaps the food being tested has proteins similar to those in pollens, and the person has developed new or stronger pollen allergies.

Maybe there are exposures to the food that are not triggering reactions beyond heightening the immune response. But we know that, at least for some people, exposures do not result in increases in the test result. In summary, an increase in a test result may not be traceable to a lack of strict avoidance of the food.

Component Tests / Molecular Diagnostics

What is component testing?

A food is made up of many different proteins that may have varying effects on allergy outcomes. Component testing separates the different proteins in a single food and measures IgE against the separate proteins. This type of testing holds promise for improved accuracy but has not been worked out for most foods. Because this method evaluates IgE against different protein molecules in a food, it is sometimes called "molecular diagnostics."

How does component testing work?

Recall that every food is a collection of proteins, and each protein may differ in being a potent or less potent allergen. Component testing separately measures IgE responses to the various proteins in a single food rather than as a mixture. For example, peanuts would no longer be thought of as one item to be tested but would rather be approached as a collection of proteins, with allergic responses to each individual protein having potential meaning. A person whose immune system recognizes (creates antibodies against) only the peanut proteins that are easily digested may be less likely to have a severe reaction than a person whose system recognizes proteins that are resistant to digestion and more likely to enter the bloodstream.

What component tests are available?

There is a small list of "approved" component tests that are widely available. Some are still being evaluated for inclusion as approved tests. Table 3.2 lists approved and emerging component tests, features of them, and possible interpretation (reviewed in Foong et al.; see chapter 11).

Table 3.2. Examples of Approved and Emerging Food Component Tests

Food	Component Tests	About the Test	Value above Which Allergy May Be Very Likely* (kU$_A$/L)
Brazil nut	Ber e 1	A potent protein	
Cashew	Ana o 3		2
Egg	Ovomucoid	Most potent protein (more than ovalbumin)	4 for regular egg (scrambled)
			50 for egg as an ingredient in bakery goods
Hazelnut	Cor a 1	Not a potent protein[†]	
	Cor a 8	A potent protein	
	Cor a 9	A potent protein	2
	Cor a 14	A potent protein	2
Milk	Casein	Most potent protein (more than whey)	5
Peanut	Ara h 1	A potent protein	
	Ara h 2	The most potent protein	2
	Ara h 3	A potent protein	
	Ara h 6	As potent as Ara h 2	
	Ara h 8	Not a potent protein[†]	
	Ara h 9	Potent but more relevant to Mediterranean geography	
Sesame	Ses i 1	A potent protein	
Soy	Gly m 8	A potent protein	2
Walnut	Jug r 1	A potent protein	
	Jug r 3	A potent protein	
Wheat	Tri a 19	A potent protein	0.5

*Very rough guide based on few studies.

[†]The protein is related to birch tree pollen.

What do we learn from component testing to peanut?

Commercial tests can measure responses to proteins called Ara h 1, 2, 3, 6, 8, and 9. Ara h 1, 2, 3, and 9 are resistant to digestion and are the "trouble-maker" proteins associated with having allergic reactions. But Ara h 2 or 6 appears to be the best indicator for peanut allergy. In contrast, Ara h 8 is digested easily and is related to protein in birch tree pollen. If the component testing is ONLY positive to Ara h 8, there may be no peanut allergy or just a mild one. In other words, a "regular" peanut skin test or blood test may be positive, and we would not know that the only reason it is positive is because of allergy to the relatively "innocent" birch pollen–related protein. The component test helps to sort this out. But the full story is more complicated. The degree of positive test also counts. So a higher test result to Ara h 2 is associated with a greater chance of peanut allergy than a lower test result. And having positive tests to several of the troublemaker proteins may also increase the chance of a true allergy compared to having responses to fewer.

What do we learn from component testing to hazelnut?

The typical hazelnut allergy blood test is very sensitive to detecting innocent allergy to birch pollen–related proteins. That is, almost everyone with a birch tree pollen protein allergy tests "positive" to the hazelnut. Some may experience an itchy mouth when eating hazelnuts, but a severe reaction is unlikely. Component testing to hazelnut separates the relatively innocent birch pollen–related protein (called Cor a 1) from other proteins that are associated with more significant allergic reactions (called Cor a 8, 9, and 14).

Does the component testing predict severity of an allergy?

Somewhat. As explained previously, the degree of positive test more accurately reflects risk of allergy than the severity of a reaction because there are additional factors that influence severity, such as state of health, having asthma, and the amount of the food eaten. Studies have conflicting findings about whether component testing reflects severity. In a rough way, increasingly strong positive tests to the potent component proteins may correspond to a higher chance for a severe reaction, or having a reaction to smaller portions of the food.

What other foods can be tested by components?

Tests like the one explained above for peanut and hazelnut are already on the market for many foods, including eggs, milk, wheat, soy, tree nuts, fruits, and vegetables. Yet most of these tests have not yet been extensively studied. Nonetheless, allergists are increasingly using such tests to provide additional insights into the nature of an individual's food allergy.

Elimination Diets

What is an elimination diet?

An elimination diet is a prescribed diet that removes one or more suspected foods from what a person eats to determine whether the food or foods are contributing to an illness.

What illnesses might be tested with an elimination diet?

Any illness that could be attributed to foods, whether the problem is allergy or any other adverse effect, could be evaluated. Typical allergic diseases that might be addressed are atopic dermatitis and chronic gastrointestinal symptoms. Elimination diets might also be used to evaluate links between foods and problems that are not considered food allergy symptoms, such as headaches, behavior, and fatigue.

Can a mother undertake an elimination diet to test her breastfed infant?

Yes, but this must be done with careful attention to the mother's nutrition. In this situation, the mother might avoid eggs or milk, for example, to see if her infant's atopic dermatitis (allergic eczema) improves.

How long does one do an elimination diet?

Typically from a week to several weeks, which is the time frame in which chronic symptoms would be expected to resolve if the appropriate trigger were removed from the diet.

Can an elimination diet be dangerous or cause allergic problems?

Yes, in an unusual way. When a food that might be causing a chronic allergic symptom when eaten consistently is removed for an extended period (weeks or months), reintroduction might trigger a sudden and sometimes severe allergic reaction. This was first noted among children suffering from atopic dermatitis who had foods to which they tested positive removed from their diets. When they retried the food, usually months later, some experienced anaphylaxis.

Why would avoiding a tolerated food sometimes lead to becoming allergic to it?

We think the immune system may maintain a balance, with mild symptoms, while the food is eaten regularly but becomes hyperreactive during a period of no exposure. This is an uncommon risk, but it must be considered when foods to which there is a positive test are removed from the diet for extended periods.

Can elimination diets carry nutritional consequences?

Elimination diets are usually brief, so nutritional deficits are uncommon. If many foods are eliminated for long periods, however, working with a dietitian to ensure nutritional adequacy may be required.

How does one decide what foods to eliminate in an elimination diet?

The foods are typically selected on the basis of personal medical history, clues from epidemiologic studies showing common triggers, and test results.

What is an example of an elimination diet?

The allergist might devise a diet that avoids all major allergens and thus excludes milk, eggs, wheat, soy, peanuts, tree nuts, fish, and shellfish. Or the doctor might create a diet that excludes one or more specific foods that are possible culprits. Or the doctor might prescribe a diet that has specified low-risk foods, such as a diet of chicken, rice, sweet potatoes, corn, apples, broccoli, string beans, and a calcium-fortified hypoallergenic drink.

What are the pitfalls of elimination diets for food allergy diagnosis?

One pitfall of the elimination diet is that the actual trigger may be left in the diet. Additionally, some chronic diseases have natural ups and downs in symptoms, so it may be confusing to determine whether the new elimination diet is responsible for symptom improvement. Finally, elimination diets are hard, and people may be apt to see improvement for all their hard work when the underlying problem is not really different—a placebo effect.

How are individual foods identified as problematic in elimination diets?
If symptoms improve after several foods are removed, it would be unclear which of the foods was responsible. Removing one at a time, although more time consuming, would more likely identify an individual trigger. Another means to identify a specific food trigger is to add one food back at a time, after symptoms have resolved to see if symptoms return. This is called an oral food challenge, or a feeding test. The oral food challenge is more definitive and can be used to address the placebo effect described above.

What is an elemental diet?
An elemental diet is one in which nutrition is provided solely by a formula that contains no whole protein, called an amino acid–based formula. In this diet, nothing being ingested could be an allergen.

Why would an elemental diet be prescribed?
This extreme diet is a definitive way to know if food is contributing to chronic symptoms. If the symptoms continue on an elemental diet, then food is not a cause.

What are the pitfalls of an elemental diet for food allergy diagnosis?
The elemental diet is extremely difficult to maintain unless it is being undertaken in an infant. People do not manage well taking no foods. Additionally, amino acid–based formulas do not taste good, although there are various flavors. Sometimes this diet is given by a feeding tube. Otherwise, pitfalls include some of the same ones that affect elimination diets, described previously. The elemental diet, however, is not plagued by the possibility that an allergen was left in the diet.

Oral Food Challenges (Feeding Tests)

What is a food challenge or feeding test?
This is a test in which a food is eaten in gradually increasing amounts under medical supervision to monitor for any symptoms, usually after the food has been eliminated from the diet for a period. The test is usually referred to as an oral food challenge.

Who does a food challenge?
Typically, an allergist suggests and supervises it.

Why is a food challenge done?
To determine whether an allergy exists or has resolved. The test is not usually undertaken just to see how severe an allergy may be. The goal of a food challenge is being able to add the food back to the diet to be enjoyed frequently.

Which types of food allergies can be tested with an oral food challenge?
Any food and any type of allergy can be tested.

Can a food challenge be used to evaluate reactions to foods that are not allergic, such as behavior problems or headaches?
Yes. The oral food challenge is a "real-world" test that can be used to evaluate the relationship of foods to any symptoms, even those not attributed to allergy, such as behavior problems, fatigue, or headaches. The test might be designed differently depending on the circumstances being evaluated. If you believe that eating a food for several days causes headaches or hyperactivity, then the test would be designed to mimic this situation.

How does the doctor decide that a food challenge is needed?
If the medical history and the test results are insufficient to confirm an allergy, the oral food challenge can be offered to make a definitive diagnosis.

What is an example of a situation that warrants a food challenge?
Let's say a child had a reaction to eggs three years ago, and at the time the skin test was 5 millimeters and the blood test was 10 kU_A/L. Now the skin test is 3 millimeters, and the blood test is 2 kU_A/L. These tests roughly indicate a 50% risk of her still being allergic. A feeding test would be needed to see if the allergy has resolved.

What is an example of a situation that would not warrant a food challenge?
If a child had an egg skin test of 3 millimeters and an egg IgE blood test of 2 kU_A/L, the tests themselves would indicate about a 50% risk of egg allergy. If she had hives from eating eggs last week, however, a feeding test would be unnecessary because her recent reaction is confirmed to have been an egg allergy by these test results.

What factors do I need to consider in deciding that a food challenge should be done?

The following should be considered:

- What is the chance I/my child will tolerate the food? Your allergist should discuss this with you. You may be more or less willing to undertake the test depending upon the odds of tolerating the food.
- Do I/my child want to include this food in the diet? While some may want to "just see" if there is an allergy, it is better to test foods that you plan to eat. Otherwise, years may pass and the question will come up again: Am I allergic?
- Will the food benefit me/my child nutritionally?
- Will the food benefit me/my child socially?
- Will undergoing the test add confidence? Usually, even a feeding test that causes a reaction will promote confidence in recognizing and treating a reaction, even if the food cannot ultimately be added to the diet.

Can I do a food challenge at home?

Usually not, unless your allergist is fairly certain that a trial would not result in anaphylaxis. For example, a food challenge to determine whether anaphylactic allergy to peanuts has resolved would not be undertaken at home. If the problem being evaluated is whether food dyes are causing hyperactivity, however, the feedings would more likely be undertaken for longer periods at home.

How many foods can be tested at one time during a food challenge?

Usually only a single food. Sometimes an allergist may offer to test two or more foods at the same time, for example, several types of beans. The benefit of trying several foods at once is efficiency, but if a reaction occurs, one may not know which food was responsible.

How are the foods given during a food challenge?

For evaluation of allergy, the food is given in gradually increasing amounts, usually in 10- to 30-minute intervals over about 60 to 120 minutes, aiming toward a meal-sized portion. Your allergist may opt to alter the dosing time or amounts.

What happens if a food challenge causes an allergic reaction?

The feeding is stopped and medications are given if needed.

When does the doctor stop giving portions of the food during a food challenge?

The allergist may temporarily halt the feeding if suspicious that a reaction is starting, or permanently if a reaction is definitely occurring.

What symptoms is the doctor looking for?

Any symptoms of an allergic reaction. Some are subtle and raise suspicion but may not be clear enough to confirm that a reaction is happening. For example, complaints of mild stomachache or odd tastes in the mouth may be normal or signs of anxiety. More obvious symptoms are hives. The allergist considers any symptoms when judging whether a reaction is occurring. When the food is eaten without symptoms, the test is often referred to as "negative" or "tolerated"; with symptoms, it is referred to as "positive" or "not tolerated." We try not to refer to the results as "passed" or "failed" because allergic reactions are not under the control of the individual, and the word "failed" could imply fault or blame.

Can a food challenge cause a severe allergic reaction, such as anaphylaxis?

Yes, but giving the food gradually and stopping at signs of a clear allergic reaction typically help to avoid severe symptoms. The purpose of this test is not to cause a severe allergic reaction but to determine whether the food is tolerated. It is important that the person being tested communicate any discomfort, such as stomach pain, so that dosing can be adjusted if needed, perhaps by slowing down to see if symptoms stop or progress.

How often does a reaction occur from a food challenge?

This varies greatly and depends on the risk assessment. Most allergists will see reaction rates of less than 30% to 50%.

How often is a severe reaction triggered by a food challenge test?

Although a food challenge can cause anaphylaxis, this happens infrequently. Most reactions will need treatment only with antihistamines. Severe reactions are uncommon because the food is given gradually and feeding is stopped when symptoms begin. Additionally, medications including epinephrine are given promptly, which also avoids severe reactions. The allergist performing the test must always be prepared to treat anaphylaxis. Fatality is possible but exceptionally rare. At this time, there have been two deaths attributed to the feeding tests, which have been performed across the globe for decades.

How much food is given during a food challenge?

The usual goal is a meal-sized portion of the food, prepared in the manner in which it will typically be consumed. In some cases, an allergist may trial a small amount of the food (a threshold challenge) to determine whether a person is sensitive to a very small amount. This might be done to reduce anxiety about accidental exposure to trace amounts. For example, most people with a sesame allergy who react to tahini (concentrated sesame paste) will tolerate a few sesame seeds, as there is far less protein in the scattered seeds.

Can a food challenge be completed without symptoms but the person be allergic anyway?

Yes. From 1% to 3% of the time, an oral food challenge without symptoms is followed by symptoms hours later or when the food is tried again days later. These later symptoms are unlikely to be severe. It is extremely unusual, however, for the food to cause symptoms after it has been successfully incorporated into the diet.

Can a person have symptoms during a food challenge but not be allergic?

Yes. This can happen in two main ways. Sometimes, a symptom coincidentally occurs during a food challenge. This results in falsely attributing the symptom to the food. Unfortunately, another common problem is that anxiety can result in symptoms that mimic an allergic reaction.

How can food challenges be performed with less risk of anxiety-caused false reactions?

First, you should talk to your allergist about any fears. A simple discussion can allay many of your concerns. The test itself can also be arranged in a way that reduces the chance that anxiety will affect the results. By hiding the test food in a way that masks the taste, and including placebo foods that do not contain the tested allergen but look, smell, and taste the same, it is easier to avoid false conclusions. The best way to accomplish this is by performing a double-blind, placebo-controlled oral food challenge.

What is involved with a double-blind, placebo-controlled oral food challenge?

In this test, a third party prepares the food. The test food is hidden in other foods to mask the taste, and a similar-tasting meal without the allergen is prepared as a placebo. The two meals are otherwise indistinguishable. They are fed in a random order under medical supervision, with neither the medical personnel nor the person being tested knowing which is which. This provides an unbiased setting for everyone involved. After the test is completed, the meal with the allergen is revealed. For example, egg powder may be hidden in one hamburger and not the other. In the morning, one hamburger is gradually eaten, and in the afternoon the other is ingested. Symptoms are recorded at each feeding and compared. If successful, these feedings are followed by eating the food in its usual form, such as scrambled eggs in this example.

What do I need to do to prepare for a food challenge?

Food challenges are usually undertaken on an empty stomach at a time when you are generally healthy. It is possible to have a light meal if there is going to be a delay. Antihistamines should not be used prior to the test for the number of days necessary for their effect to be lost, which varies according to the type of antihistamine. Other allergy and asthma medications can be continued. The testing cannot be performed if asthma or eczema flare up on the day of scheduled testing, so these should be kept under control. Talk to your doctor if you have ongoing symptoms that might interfere with the food challenge. Be sure to discuss the risks and benefits of the tests with your allergist. You should also bring your emergency medications with you for the food challenge. Your doctor will have the medications available, but this way you will have treatments in the unlikely event that symptoms occur after you have left the office or hospital.

How can children prepare for a food challenge?

Explain to children that they might not be allergic to the food and that this test is necessary to find out if they can eat it. Explain that they might experience an allergic reaction, but if they do, the symptoms are usually mild and will be treated with medications. Let children know that this is an exception to the usual rule, that it is okay for them to try the food to which they may be allergic. Consider bringing toys, games, and appropriate distractions. Discuss with your doctor whether you should bring foods that the child enjoys that contain the allergen. Consider bringing favorite utensils and dishes to provide familiarity.

How long should one wait before having another food challenge to the same food if it was not tolerated the first time?

This depends on the food, the test results, the features of the reaction, personal preferences, and other factors. Typically, allergists wait at least a year between challenges to the same food.

What happens if the test causes an allergic reaction?

You will be instructed to continue avoiding the food. This is a disappointing outcome, but many people take comfort in having a confirmed reason to continue avoiding the food, rather than just an assumption that they have an allergy. Sometimes people also learn about the amount of food that triggers a reaction and the kinds of symptoms to expect, which can be helpful for practical reasons in daily living. For example, there may be less anxiety about trace amounts of exposure if an entire serving caused only a mild symptom.

Can an allergic reaction during a food challenge make the allergy worse or last longer?

Probably not. There are not sufficient studies on this, but in my study of children undergoing feeding tests to milk and egg, we did not see a "boosting" of allergy test results after reactions during food challenges. We also studied children who had one-time accidental exposures and reactions to milk, egg, or peanut and similarly did not see a boosting of allergy tests. Additionally, there are those who almost tolerate the feeding test the first time and then fully tolerate the test the next year.

What happens if the test reveals that the food is tolerated?

In this case, the food should be added back as a regular part of the diet. Let your doctor know if you have any suspicion that the food is causing a problem. Be careful to avoid other foods you are allergic to when purchasing new foods that contain the now acceptable ingredient.

Can a food allergy return after tolerating the food during a food challenge?

It is possible to develop an allergy to any food at any age, so having a recurrence of an allergy is a theoretical possibility. Recurrence of an allergy after tolerating the food during an oral food challenge, however, is uncommon. It has happened with peanut allergies, but almost all individuals who reported recurrence after tolerating peanut during a challenge test had not incorporated peanuts into their diets. Their symptoms occurred when they tried peanuts again about a year following the successful food challenge. In contrast, it appears that those who did incorporate peanuts into their diets did not experience these problems. This is why it is suggested to eat the food regularly after a successful ingestion test. It is important to recognize that this recommendation applies to children who clearly had an allergy and the allergy resolved, rather than to children who simply never ate a particular food and were tested to determine whether their positive test indicated an allergy.

How often does the food have to be eaten after an oral food challenge determines it is tolerated?

There is no specific regimen for incorporating the food. Including it in the diet should not be stressful. Simply ingest the food periodically, as one would do naturally, and don't avoid it any longer.

What are the possible emotional consequences of a food challenge test?

You would probably think that a reaction during the test would lead to sadness and increased anxiety, but studies have shown that even this outcome is typically associated with improved quality of life. When people know that they are avoiding a food for a good reason and have faced the potential unknown of what a reaction is like, they often feel empowered. Everyone is different, however, and you should discuss how a reaction during the test might affect you or your child. Sometimes professional mental health counseling is needed before or after a food challenge to reduce anxiety.

Additional Tests

What is a food patch test?

This test is performed by placing the food on the skin, usually under a small metal cap, for a day or two. Two or three days after removal, the area is checked for rash.

Why would a food patch test be performed?

Food patch tests have been used to evaluate illnesses that might not produce immediate allergic reactions as well as illnesses in which IgE antibodies to the food are not produced. These conditions include eosinophilic esophagitis, food protein–induced enterocolitis syndrome, and atopic dermatitis (eczema). The theory is that these delayed allergic reactions on the skin patch test may reflect the chronic or delayed reactions of these illnesses.

Is the food patch test painful?

No, but it can be itchy and uncomfortable. It is sometimes difficult to keep a test in place because of irritation and sweating.

Can a food patch test cause a severe reaction?

Having a food touch the skin is not likely to result in severe reactions.

Is the food patch test accurate?

The accuracy of the test has been disproven for food protein–induced enterocolitis, and the diagnostic benefit remains uncertain for other food-related illnesses.

Is the food patch test a routinely performed food allergy test?

No. It is not studied well enough to be considered a standard or routine allergy test.

What is a test for total IgE?

A test for total IgE measures all IgE antibodies in the bloodstream. Total IgE does not give any specific diagnostic information. Sometimes allergists perform this test to get a relative idea of the proportion of food-specific IgE because if the total IgE is very high, it could cast suspicion that food-specific results may be "inflated" and less predictive of allergy. But studies have so far not proven that determining total IgE reliably assists in diagnosing a specific food allergy.

What is an intradermal test?

An intradermal test is a skin test that is performed by injecting a small amount of extract into the skin, rather than simply scratching or pricking it. This method is not recommended because it is too likely to result in positive results that are meaningless (known as a false positive), and it carries the risk of causing a generalized allergic reaction.

Unproven and Disproven Tests

What tests are not considered helpful?

Several tests are considered unproven and are not recommended by food allergy experts. These include applied kinesiology, provocation-neutralization, resistance testing, cytotoxic testing, and IgG/IgG4 testing.

What is applied kinesiology?

An applied kinesiology test has the individual hold a food, which is often in a glass bottle, while muscle strength is being checked, with a notion that weakness indicates an allergy. There is no clear scientific basis for the test. When this method was subject to blinding (hiding the bottle contents from the practitioner), the results varied, indicating that some degree of suggestion or bias is likely at work when this testing is performed.

What is provocation-neutralization?

The food is given in small amounts (doses) that increase until symptoms are provoked (provocation), and then a lower dose is given to stop the symptoms (neutralization). This is usually done by mouth, but sometimes by injection. The symptoms tested are usually subjective (fatigue, drowsiness, skin itch, pain, chills, stomach upset, and so forth) and not typical of allergies. About fifteen studies looked at the effectiveness of this approach, but only eight were done without the provider knowing the doses and substances, and only one was done with a comparison group. Several of the studies showed poor results, including a 70% rate of improvement using false treatments. In one widely publicized study that was properly performed, with the testing blinded and a comparison group included, provocation-neutralization was not effective (using salt water had the same result as using the treatment extracts). It seems that the approach relies on the placebo effect and the suggestion of improvement from the person doing the test.

What is VEGA, or resistance testing?

Electronic equipment measures the flow of electricity through the body, with the idea that variations indicate a potential allergy. The person being tested holds the food in hand or on an aluminum plate. Sometimes the testing is done for a child by testing the parent, who holds the child's hand. A computer makes readouts of the results. A controlled study showed no difference in results between people with or without allergies. There is no reason to expect this test to be useful, and there is no proof that it is helpful. For example, there are additional electronic systems that claim to use laser technology, which remains unproven.

What is IgG/IgG4 testing?

IgG, or IgG4, are antibodies (proteins) that can recognize food proteins. Although tests are sold to measure these antibodies, having them does not appear to correlate with specific allergies. In fact, in studies attempting to treat food allergies, these antibodies appear to increase when the treatment is going well. Additionally, individuals who do not react to foods have these antibodies. Therefore these tests are not recommended to diagnose a food allergy. Their role in monitoring resolution of food allergies is under study.

What is hair analysis?

Hair is analyzed to somehow determine allergies. Laboratories claiming to be able to diagnose allergies this way were put to the test decades ago and failed. Body chemical analysis is a related test where blood or other body fluids are tested for various chemicals. Anyone can have these chemicals in their bodies, and a relation to allergy is not known or proven.

What is a pulse test?

Checking the pulse to measure response to a food was suggested in the 1940s. One might guess that the pulse would change during a severe allergic reaction, but the test has no dependable diagnostic value.

What are cytotoxic testing and ALCAT?

Both tests measure cell responses to foods. Cytotoxic testing looks at cell death under a microscope, and the ALCAT test measures the size of cells as a reflection of their activity. There is no strong scientific rationale behind these tests nor large-scale studies supporting their use.

Why do people undergo tests that traditional allergists and expert panels recommend against?

These tests have failed to pass scientific rigor, but they are not outlawed. Unfortunately, "buyer beware" is the current situation with allergy testing.

How can I learn more about whether to trust various tests?

I like Dr. Stephen Barrett's website, appropriately titled Quackwatch (www .quackwatch.com).

Improved Diagnostic Tests

What is on the horizon for improved diagnostic tests?

The goal of improved food allergy diagnostic testing is to have tests that can predict allergies more accurately and provide insights into severity, threshold, response to therapies, and prognosis.

What is a basophil activation test?

A basophil activation test is a laboratory test in which a food is mixed with allergy cells to see if the cells respond. This is similar to a skin test, except that it is performed in a test tube. This test shows some significant promise but is still not routinely performed. It does not work in about 10% of people and requires technical lab work that is just now starting to be automated in a way that may allow commercialization. A similar test using a similar cell (the mast cell) is also under study.

What could the basophil activation test offer?

Preliminary studies suggest it may help to identify the amount of food that could trigger a reaction or reaction severity, but much more testing is needed.

What is epitope testing?

Every food protein has various areas on it that the immune system might recognize. The exact areas recognized may reflect different risks of having an allergic response. For example, a child making IgE antibodies to segments of a single milk protein that survives digestion may be less likely to outgrow milk allergy and more prone to severe reactions than a child whose IgE antibodies recognize only segments of milk protein that do not survive digestion. Studies have been promising, and commercialization of epitope testing is just starting. VeriMAP is a new peanut allergy diagnostic test that uses epitopes. These tests are undergoing additional research to determine their place in diagnosis.

What is affinity testing?

The strength with which the IgE attaches to protein—its "affinity"—may influence the severity or persistence of an allergy. The stronger the attachment, the more likely the allergy will be severe or persistent. More studies are needed to investigate this possibility, but early studies have shown promise in using this approach to distinguish children with transient or persistent milk allergy.

What else is on the horizon for improved diagnostics?

There are many new methods being evaluated. There are attempts at "miniaturization" of standard tests so that less blood is needed. Studies are looking at how cells respond in the test tube, at gene activation, at the production of various chemicals, and at other cell responses. There is also interest in looking at the pattern of chemicals in the blood, assessing multiple different immune responses all at once, and using a "supercomputer" approach to assess many different tests (including the medical history) at the same time to come up with a best-guess diagnosis using all available data. The eventual goal is to reduce the need for feeding tests.

Chapter Lessons

Rachel, who is now 10 years old, had an allergic reaction consisting of hives when she ate peanut at age 2. She had a small positive skin test to peanut at the time, and over the years her peanut skin test caused a reaction that grew larger in area. She had blood tests to peanut that also increased over time: age 2 years, 3 kU_A/L; age 4 years, 7 kU_A/L; age 6 years, 10 kU_A/L; and age 8 years, 14 kU_A/L. Over these years she never ate peanut. She developed hay fever. She and her family were upset that her peanut allergy had persisted.

When she came to me with these records, I took note of the fact that over the years she had developed hay fever. I tested her to birch pollen, discovering a large positive skin prick test. Knowing that peanut has "innocent" birch pollen–related proteins, I ordered component testing to peanut that revealed the only positive test was to Ara h 8, the pollen-related protein. I had Rachel undergo a food challenge to peanut butter, and although she had a slight itchy mouth at first, she completed a full feeding with no symptoms and was able to add peanut back into her diet.

This case illustrates that the peanut allergy tests were likely increasing only because of Rachel's increasing pollen allergy, while she was in fact losing her allergy to the "troublemaker" proteins in peanut. The peanut component tests are valuable in evaluating this possibility. We also see that she had a slight mouth itch during the test, which is not uncommon when there is a strong pollen allergy. It was important to have a medically supervised feeding test in Rachel's situation because she certainly had a prior peanut allergy, and sometimes (rarely) the component tests to Ara h 1, 2, 3, and 9 are negative but still a reaction happens. She will be encouraged to make peanut a routine part of her diet to reduce the risk of recurrence of peanut allergy, a problem that happens more often when a person who outgrew peanut allergy strictly avoids peanut despite tolerating it during a feeding test.

Paul is an 18-month-old with severe eczema. His parents thought the rash might be worse with eggs. His pediatrician sent blood tests with the following results: egg, 10 kU_A/L; milk, 5 kU_A/L; wheat, 45 kU_A/L; soy, 17 kU_A/L; peanut 2 kU_A/L; corn, 34 kU_A/L. They removed all of these foods from the diet and noticed minimal improvement in the rash. They saw me with these tests in hand and said they needed to see me because Paul is allergic to "everything."

I explained that the most important test is Paul's life story and that I wanted to hear it. I learned that Paul was a great eater and had a varied diet up until the testing was done the prior month. He ate all of the foods that were tested. They never bothered him, but the family had learned that eczema could be related to foods and then thought he had some worse days when he ate egg. After discussing this more, however, it became apparent that his eczema, like usual eczema, had ups and downs. His pediatrician had ordered a "panel" of tests without consideration of the history. I explained how many people have positive tests but can eat the foods anyway. Removing foods for no good reason can have nutritional, social, and even allergy ramifications, as avoidance of tolerated foods in the face of positive tests can sometimes result in new, even severe, allergies to previously tolerated foods.

Given that Paul had only avoided the foods for a few weeks, I had the family gradually restart all of them, and he did fine. Some changes in his skin care regimen further helped his rashes.

CHAPTER 4

Recognizing and Treating Anaphylaxis

Anaphylaxis is a severe allergic reaction. Understanding the symptoms and treatments is essential to protect yourself and others from this most dangerous type of food allergy reaction. In this chapter, I answer questions about anaphylaxis symptoms and treatments.

General Questions about Anaphylaxis

What is anaphylaxis?

Anaphylaxis is a severe allergic reaction that is rapid in onset and can be fatal. Symptoms occur beyond where the food has made contact, beyond the mouth and gut. Typically, several areas of the body are affected, for example, the skin and the gut, or the gut and breathing.

What is anaphylactic shock?

When anaphylaxis leads to poor blood circulation that deprives the body of oxygen and nutrients, it is called "shock."

What foods cause anaphylaxis?

Any food can potentially cause anaphylaxis, but the ones that do so most often are peanuts, tree nuts, shellfish, fish, milk, and eggs.

Who is at risk of anaphylaxis?

Anyone could develop a food allergy that results in anaphylaxis. The risks of food anaphylaxis are the same as those for food allergy: having a family or personal history of allergic problems, such as asthma, atopic dermatitis

Table 4.1. Symptoms of Anaphylaxis

Part of the Body / Organ System	Symptoms
Skin	Many hives (look like mosquito bites), itchy redness over the body, swelling (such as of the eyes or lips)
Breathing*	Shortness of breath, wheezing, chest tightness, repetitive coughing, throat tightness, hoarseness, trouble breathing or swallowing, drooling, obstructive swelling of the tongue
Gut	Vomiting, cramping pain, diarrhea (when combined with other symptoms)
Circulation*	Pale or blue skin, faintness, weak pulse, dizziness, confusion
Other	Feeling of "impending doom," uterine contractions

*Individual symptoms that suggest a severe reaction.

(eczema), hay fever, or food allergies. Allergies to foods that more often cause severe reactions—namely, peanuts, tree nuts, fish, and shellfish—may represent an increased risk. Persons with coexisting asthma appear to have a higher risk of more severe food-allergic reactions.

What are the symptoms of anaphylaxis?
No specific symptom defines anaphylaxis. Symptoms might occur in any of several body areas (systems) and may involve various symptoms in each of them. Table 4.1 lists symptoms of anaphylaxis.

How long after eating a food can anaphylaxis happen?
From minutes to about two hours. It is rare for symptoms to begin more than two hours after the food was eaten, and unusual for them to begin more than an hour afterward. Most of the time, symptoms begin within 20 minutes of ingesting the trigger food.

What pattern of symptoms would definitely be anaphylaxis?
There is no single pattern. An itchy mouth, few hives, or isolated gut symptoms would not qualify as anaphylaxis, but combinations of symptoms would. Therefore a person with hives and vomiting from a food-allergic reaction is experiencing anaphylaxis. A severe symptom after a food is

eaten could qualify as anaphylaxis even if it is the only symptom. For example, a person with poor blood circulation after ingesting a food allergen is experiencing anaphylaxis.

If there are no hives, can one assume anaphylaxis is not occurring?

No. It is possible to have anaphylaxis without any skin symptoms. Knowing this is VERY important because fatalities have been attributed to ignoring treatment of anaphylaxis for lack of seeing a rash.

Are there specific symptoms during anaphylaxis that are dangerous?

Yes. Any symptoms affecting breathing or circulation are serious. Breathing symptoms include shortness of breath, wheezing, chest tightness, repetitive coughing, throat tightness, hoarseness, trouble breathing or swallowing, drooling, and obstructive swelling of the tongue. Blood circulation symptoms include pale or blue skin, confusion, and passing out. A feeling of "impending doom" can also precede serious symptoms.

What are the milder symptoms during anaphylaxis?

Skin rashes and swelling, mouth itch, sneezing and nose symptoms, and gut symptoms are not intrinsically dangerous.

Besides foods, what else triggers anaphylaxis?

Triggers include medications, insect stings, vaccinations, latex, and anaphylaxis for no clear reason, called idiopathic anaphylaxis.

Are there illnesses that mimic anaphylaxis?

There are several. Among them are scombroid fish poisoning (spoilage of dark-meat fish that releases histamine-like toxins), panic attacks, choking, heart attacks, and allergic responses such as asthma or hives.

How can one tell an asthma attack from anaphylaxis?

It may be tricky. Asthma triggers include viral infections, exercise, cold air, and inhalation of allergens, such as pollens or animal dander. Isolated wheezing after these triggers is most likely asthma. Asthma symptoms of cough and wheeze without other symptoms, such as itchy mouth or hives, and without a known or likely exposure to a food allergen are most likely due to an asthma flare.

What should you do if you are not sure a reaction is truly anaphylaxis or another medical problem?

If there is a suspicion of anaphylaxis, it is best to treat a person for it. In all cases, administer first-aid management and activate emergency health care responses, for example, by calling 911.

How long does anaphylaxis last?

In most cases, the anaphylactic reaction lasts less than an hour when treated appropriately. Sometimes symptoms return over the subsequent hours. Rarely, anaphylaxis symptoms can continue in waves for days.

How often does anaphylaxis occur in more than one wave of symptoms?

It depends on the severity of the first wave of symptoms. If the first wave was mild, a second wave is less likely to occur. Studies have estimated that a second wave occurs in 1% to 20% of reactions. Sometimes the second wave is more severe.

What is the timing of additional waves of symptoms during anaphylaxis?

If additional waves of symptoms occur at all, they usually happen within a few hours of the onset of the reaction. It is therefore recommended to stay under medical supervision for at least four hours after a reaction has subsided. This instruction would vary based on the severity of the reaction, for example, longer if serious symptoms occurred.

How quickly can an allergic reaction progress from mild to severe?

Within minutes. Progression of symptoms can also occur over hours, however.

How do I know when anaphylaxis is going to happen?

Unfortunately, it is not predictable.

Why do I need to understand how to recognize anaphylaxis?

Because prompt treatment is needed to address the symptoms adequately.

How often is anaphylaxis fatal?

Rarely, but the risk is greater if treatment is delayed. Of course, any death from a food allergy is a senseless death. Scientific reports in 2013 by

Umasunthar et al. and in 2018 by Pouessel et al. (see chapter 11) looked at the world literature on fatal food anaphylaxis and estimated minimum rates of 3 per 100 million annually. The authors tried to put the allergy-related death rates into context. Considering children from birth to age 19 with food allergy, the risk of a fatal food-allergic reaction was greater than the risk of dying from a lightning strike, a bit less likely than death due to fire, about one-tenth as likely as death due to murder, and less than one-hundredth as likely as death due to other causes.

What are the risks for fatal food anaphylaxis?

Studies of people who died from allergic reactions revealed the main factors they seemed to share and the presumed reasons these factors are risks. The risk factors for fatal reactions include

• delaying treatment with epinephrine
• being a teenager or young adult
• having asthma
• having a diagnosed food allergy
• having a history of reactions to trace exposures
• having the reaction away from home
• not having hives during the fatal episode
• being allergic to peanuts, tree nuts, fish, shellfish, or milk

Why is delayed treatment with epinephrine a risk for fatal food anaphylaxis?

Epinephrine is the most crucial treatment for anaphylaxis. Waiting too long may make treatment less effective. In one study of children and teens with severe food-allergic reactions, the ones who survived received epinephrine within about 15 minutes after symptoms began, whereas those who died did not receive treatment until about an hour after symptoms began.

Why are teenagers and young adults at greater risk for fatal food anaphylaxis?

Presumably, these are individuals who are more likely to eat risky foods, to not carry their medications, and to not treat their symptoms promptly.

Why is having coexisting asthma a risk for fatal food anaphylaxis?

It is believed that having asthma, or "twitchy airways," makes the airways more vulnerable to becoming reactive during a food-allergic reaction. Therefore a person with asthma who experiences an allergic reaction to a food is more likely to have breathing difficulties during the reaction, which is a severe symptom.

Why is having a previously diagnosed food allergy a risk for fatal food anaphylaxis?

We do not know exactly. Although a first allergic reaction is occasionally fatal, most who have succumbed had a known allergy.

Why is having a history of reactions to trace exposures a risk for fatal food anaphylaxis?

Those who are more sensitive may be at higher risk.

Why is having a reaction away from home a risk for fatal food anaphylaxis?

Presumably, being in unfamiliar settings or not having access to medications can be a risk, which is why education about avoidance and always having a prescribed treatment available are so important.

Why is a lack of hives during anaphylaxis associated with fatal outcomes?

Many people erroneously believe that anaphylaxis must include hives. This assumption may lead to delayed treatment. It is essential to understand that anaphylaxis can occur without hives (about 20% of the time).

Why are anaphylactic reactions to peanuts, tree nuts, fish, shellfish, and milk associated with fatal outcomes?

These are the foods most often associated with severe reactions, although any food can trigger anaphylaxis. Peanuts and tree nuts account for the majority of fatal reactions.

How does one prevent fatal anaphylaxis?

By avoiding the trigger and seeking prompt treatment.

What should be done for a person having anaphylaxis?

Prompt treatment with epinephrine and alerting emergency medical care, for example, by calling 911.

When calling 911 about food anaphylaxis, what should the dispatcher be told?

The 911 dispatcher should be told that the person is experiencing anaphylaxis, whatever treatments were given, and how they are doing. Some states do not automatically have allergy treatments available on ambulances, so explaining the situation may ensure that the correct emergency unit is dispatched, one that has medications such as epinephrine.

Why go to an emergency room for anaphylaxis?

A person who is experiencing anaphylaxis should be taken to an emergency room for evaluation and possibly additional treatments that are available there. An emergency room is preferable to a doctor's office because the office is less likely to be well equipped to treat a progressive reaction.

How long should a person who experienced anaphylaxis stay in an emergency room?

At least four hours to be observed for recurrence of symptoms. The observation period might be longer if the symptoms were severe or continued to occur.

My doctor told me to always go to an emergency room if I inject epinephrine. Why?

Many people erroneously think that injecting epinephrine is itself the reason to go to an emergency room, as if the epinephrine might cause a medical problem. I worry that this MISCONCEPTION can make a person reluctant to inject the epinephrine! The reason you should go to an emergency room after injecting epinephrine is not about the epinephrine. The reason is that you experienced a serious allergic reaction that needs to be monitored in case symptoms worsen or recur.

Do I always have to go the emergency room if I experienced anaphylaxis?

The COVID-19 pandemic brought up the question: If my emergency room is overflowing with sick patients, and I am worried I could get sick, do I still have to go there for anaphylaxis? As mentioned above, the advice to go to an emergency room is about careful monitoring in case symptoms are not responding or return. Some experts recommended staying home if the symptoms responded well to epinephrine. This judgment call involves thinking about the individual person's risk of developing progressively severe symptoms compared to the risk of being in the emergency department (which would be high only in extreme circumstances). Never delay injecting epinephrine because of a concern about access to an emergency room.

What plans should be in place for a person at risk of anaphylaxis?

A person who is at risk for food anaphylaxis should be prescribed self-injectable epinephrine, be encouraged to carry their medications, be trained in how and when to use it, and be educated about allergen avoidance.

Are there any situations that increase a person's risk for food anaphylaxis? What are cofactors or augmentation factors?

For a person with a food allergy, several circumstances might increase the risk of a more severe or anaphylactic allergic reaction, including eating a larger amount of the food, exercising, taking aspirin or alcohol, having a viral illness, and menstruating.

What is the relationship between exercise, food, and anaphylaxis?

Some people can eat a specific food or foods and have no symptoms unless they exercise near the time of the meal. This problem is called food-associated exercise-induced anaphylaxis (FAEIA). Sometimes any food will cause this problem, but more often specific ones do. The most common triggers are wheat, celery, and seafood. Treatment requires avoidance of the food for at least four hours prior to exercise. A person with FAEIA should always exercise with a buddy and have anaphylaxis treatments on hand. In addition, eating a food to which you are allergic and then exercising may increase the severity of a reaction.

What are the theories about why food-associated exercise-induced anaphylaxis happens?

One theory to explain FAEIA is that exercise may alter gut blood flow, allowing certain proteins to be absorbed more readily into the bloodstream. Another theory is that exercise activates gut enzymes that may alter proteins in a way that makes them more visible to the immune system, resulting in reactions.

How do aspirin and alcohol increase the risk of food anaphylaxis?

Most likely by making the stomach lining more prone to quickly absorb food allergens into the bloodstream.

How does a viral illness or menstruation increase the risk of anaphylaxis?

It is thought that some people are susceptible to changes in their immune response during illness or menstruation, leading to a more robust allergic reaction.

What can be done to improve safety for teenagers at risk for anaphylaxis?

We think that teenagers are a high-risk group because they are more likely to eat a food without making sure it is safe and are less likely to promptly treat a reaction. Studies suggest that social reasons (peer pressure, feeling different) and possibly a teenager's feeling of invincibility are the main factors. When we asked teens about their allergies, they indicated that they wanted others to better understand food allergies. They were less likely to carry medications when they assumed there was less risk (sports, dances where food was not served) or did not have a convenient means to carry them. Based on these studies, I think it is essential for readers (especially parents, teachers, coaches, and so forth) to address the problems shown in table 4.2.

What should I be discussing with my food-allergic teenager?

Start conversations on food allergy topics well before problems (such as risk-taking) might arise. Ask your teen, "What would you do if you had a reaction at a party or with friends?" Discuss times when your teen might think it is not necessary to carry medications, and explore options to make consistent carrying easier to do. Discuss peer pressure. Discuss dating (and kissing). Discuss when epinephrine should be used. Openly discuss any resistance to self-injection. Discuss how to approach dining out with friends. Emphasize that alcohol use can result in increased risk-taking and worse reactions should an accident occur. Emphasize that independence requires increasing acceptance of responsibility. Involve your allergist in these conversations as well.

Table 4.2. Addressing Issues That Increase Risk of Fatal Anaphylaxis for Teenagers and Young Adults

Problem	Approaches
Misperception of "anaphylaxis"	• Teach the symptoms to look out for, not just the word "anaphylaxis"
Low rate of epinephrine autoinjector use	• Educate about treatment circumstances (the need to inject promptly, when to inject) • Review injector technique • Work with your doctor to make sure the teenager is comfortable and confident in using the medication
Inconsistency in carrying autoinjector, varying by social circumstances (less at parties), perceived risks (less at sporting activities), and convenience (clothing that does not have pockets)	• Impress on the teenager the need for consistency • Issue reminders to carry consistently, especially to sports and social activities • Offer alternatives that make carrying the autoinjector easier (purse, holster) • Have an autoinjector on-site when appropriate (for example, coaches, teachers)
Risky eating	• Review risks of exposures and discourage risky behavior • Supervise early practice in obtaining safe foods to instill good habits • Encourage peer education
Feeling "different" or "less concerned," leading to risk taking	• Encourage third-party education about allergies, especially for friends • Encourage peers to work together to protect the teen who has the food allergy
Difficulty in obtaining safe foods	• Increase safe food options • Assign a "point person" for safe meals (for example, in the cafeteria)

Epinephrine

What is epinephrine?

Epinephrine is a medication similar to adrenaline, which is made by the body during a "fight or flight" reaction. Epinephrine reduces swelling, opens the breathing tubes, tightens blood vessels to carry blood more effectively, and strengthens the heartbeat.

What symptoms does epinephrine treat?

Epinephrine treats all the severe symptoms of anaphylaxis, reducing throat swelling and wheezing and improving blood circulation.

How is epinephrine given?

By injection.

Who should be prescribed epinephrine?

Anyone who is at risk for anaphylaxis.

How is it determined that a person is at risk for food anaphylaxis?

Your doctor must decide whether this is the case, but epinephrine should certainly be prescribed for anyone who has already experienced severe allergic reactions to foods. Persons considered at risk may include anyone with food allergies, but especially allergies to peanuts, tree nuts, shellfish, or fish. Prescriptions of self-injectable epinephrine are usually considered for anyone who has more than a mild type of food allergy (for example, oral allergy syndrome), especially for those who also have asthma. Some physicians prescribe it even for people with milder reactions.

Where on the body is epinephrine injected?

In the middle part of the upper leg, roughly midway between the front and side.

Can the injection be given through clothing?

Yes, although it is a good idea to take a few extra seconds to pull pants down or lift up a dress to avoid hitting a seam or something in a pocket that might block the injection.

When should epinephrine be given?

Whenever anaphylaxis is occurring or is likely to develop, epinephrine should be injected promptly. As described above, combinations of symptoms in different areas of the body, or any severe symptoms after a known or likely food allergen was eaten, would indicate that anaphylaxis is occurring and warrant injection of epinephrine.

Why is it necessary to inject epinephrine promptly during anaphylaxis?

Getting the most benefit from epinephrine throughout the body requires adequate blood circulation to carry it. If one waits too long, the heart and circulation may not be able to get the medication where it is needed. Promptly receiving epinephrine for anaphylaxis is associated with a lower risk of being hospitalized and a lower risk of needing multiple doses.

Should epinephrine be given before anaphylaxis if there are allergic symptoms?

There are situations when the answer is "yes." This takes some judgment, but if a person with a known severe allergy has definitely eaten an allergen and is having allergic symptoms, it is reasonable to inject epinephrine without waiting for symptoms that indicate anaphylaxis.

Should epinephrine ever be given before any allergic symptoms develop?

The answer to this is controversial. Some experts have suggested that it may be a good decision to inject epinephrine even before any symptoms develop in specific circumstances. A situation where this might be considered is when a person definitely ingested the food allergen that has caused extremely severe allergic reactions in the past, such as near-fatal anaphylaxis. If this is done, however, one should have an additional dose of epinephrine available in case severe symptoms emerge and should activate emergency services (call 911) to get to medical care, since a reaction is likely impending. Giving an injection of epinephrine prior to developing any symptoms is not commonly recommended, and experts have increasingly advised against this practice.

What symptoms of an allergic reaction would not require epinephrine?

In general, if there are only mild symptoms—such as several hives, some stomach upset, or mouth itching—epinephrine can usually be withheld because other medications can treat the mild symptoms. There should be careful monitoring, however, to watch for any progression of symptoms that may warrant epinephrine.

How fast does epinephrine work?
Usually there is relief within minutes.

How long do the effects of epinephrine last?
The medication effects last for about 20 to 30 minutes, but usually only one dose is needed.

How often does a person need more than one dose of epinephrine?
This happens about 10% to 20% of the time. Unless prompt medical care is not available, the second dose is more often given by medical personnel at a hospital emergency room.

What would be a reason to give more than one dose of epinephrine?
If the symptoms did not respond well enough or they recur, more doses can be given.

How long should you wait before giving a second dose of epinephrine?
Guidelines state 5 to 20 minutes. But if a person is having severe trouble breathing or is not responding well because of poor blood circulation, giving another dose in less than 5 minutes may be reasonable.

How many doses of epinephrine should a food-allergic person carry?
Generally two, because a second dose might be needed.

How does an autoinjector work?
A premeasured amount of epinephrine is injected automatically.

What autoinjectors of epinephrine are available?
Various brand-name and generic epinephrine autoinjectors are currently on the market, with more in the pipeline. Some brands that have been available in the United States are EpiPen, Auvi-Q (called ALLERJECT in Canada), and Adrenaclick. Generic autoinjectors may look and work exactly like the EpiPen or Adrenaclick, or they may be an entirely different device, such as the generic autoinjector manufactured by TEVA. Additional

devices are available globally, such as Emerade and Jext. Whatever device you and your doctor decide on, or is available from your pharmacy, the crucial point to discuss is how to activate the medication. If your pharmacist dispenses a device that you are not familiar with, immediately discuss this with the pharmacist and your doctor. All of the autoinjector types have online videos, and practice trainer devices are available.

How many doses of epinephrine are in an autoinjector?
Current autoinjectors have one dose and are discarded after use.

Does epinephrine have to be injected from an autoinjector?
No. There is a prefilled injector that can be prescribed for treatment of anaphylaxis, called SYMJEPI. This device looks like a small syringe and is different from the autoinjectors because rather than being activated by pressure against the leg and automatically delivering the needle and medication, the SYMJEPI is used like a typical needle and syringe. A cover is removed, revealing the needle, and after inserting the needle into the leg, a cylinder is pressed to deliver the epinephrine. Epinephrine is also available in small glass vials from which it can be drawn into a syringe and injected by hand. Medical professionals typically use this method to give epinephrine in the hospital. Although this is an option, injecting epinephrine by syringe after taking a measured amount from a vial requires extra skill and is more prone to errors in measuring and injecting. Therefore most physicians prefer autoinjectors or prefilled syringes for first-aid treatment of anaphylaxis.

Is epinephrine always effective to treat anaphylaxis?
Epinephrine is very effective, especially when given promptly for anaphylaxis. There are reports of fatal food anaphylaxis despite appropriate treatment with epinephrine, however. This is why you should NEVER take risks with your diet by thinking that if you have a reaction, you can simply depend on the epinephrine. One reported death was of a teenager who took risks when thinking this way.

How can I learn and teach others about how to use an epinephrine autoinjector?
You should ask your doctor to demonstrate how and when to use the device, using a trainer. You can also watch videos online from the manufacturer's

website. If you have an expired device, you can practice by injecting it into an orange. But do not eat the orange! And take the expired device to your doctor or local hospital for disposal.

What if epinephrine is given but the person was not having anaphylaxis?

Epinephrine injected into the leg muscle is very safe, which is one reason it is better to use it if in doubt. Whether given to a person having anaphylaxis or not, the side effects are the same. This medication was routinely used to treat asthma before asthma inhalers became the main therapy.

Can repeated use of epinephrine make it less effective?

No. People do not become resistant to the effects of epinephrine from prior use.

What are the side effects of epinephrine?

The most common side effects are increased heart rate and some jitteriness or tremor, similar to having too much caffeine. A person may also develop a headache and appear pale or sometimes flushed.

Is epinephrine dangerous?

No. There is some risk for people with heart problems who may not tolerate a faster heart rate, but epinephrine should be injected for anaphylaxis even if there is a heart problem. Persons with a known heart condition should discuss their anaphylactic food allergy with their physician.

Can a pregnant woman receive epinephrine?

Epinephrine is safe to inject for treatment of anaphylaxis in pregnant women.

Are there any medications that should not be taken if epinephrine is prescribed?

Some medications, such as beta-blockers, could interact poorly with the epinephrine, and alternative medications to treat heart problems or high blood pressure could be chosen. Talk to your doctor about these alternatives. Because anaphylaxis is life-threatening, it is recommended to inject epinephrine for anaphylaxis even if a person has heart problems or is on medications that may interact poorly.

How long do epinephrine side effects last?

Usually for less than 30 minutes.

Do autoinjectors expire?

Yes. Always check the expiration date. When new, they should be dated for at least one year. If your pharmacist gives you one with an expiration date in less than a year, ask for a newer one.

What if I forgot to replace an expired autoinjector but that is all that I have to treat anaphylaxis?

While it would be preferable to have an unexpired autoinjector, if there is anaphylaxis and no other options, an expired autoinjector is better than not using any. There is likely to be some active medication remaining.

What should I do with my expired epinephrine autoinjector?

First, make sure you have new autoinjectors available. You can use the expired ones to practice injecting into an orange, as described above. Take the used or expired autoinjector to your doctor or local emergency room to be disposed of as medical waste.

Why does the epinephrine autoinjector have a window?

If the medication goes bad for some reason, it can become discolored with a brown hue. The window allows one to check if this has happened.

How do I store an epinephrine autoinjector?

The manufacturers generally suggest that autoinjectors be stored at room temperature, which is generally between 68 and 77 degrees Fahrenheit (20 to 25 degrees Celsius), with allowable temperature fluctuations of 59 to 86 degrees Fahrenheit (15 to 30 degrees Celsius). This is usually achieved by carrying it on your person or in a carrying pouch. If you are going to be in extremes of heat or cold, you could store the autoinjector in a cooler, a temperature-resistant pouch, or an empty thermos. Do not leave it in a glove compartment in the heat or freezing cold.

If I left an autoinjector in extreme heat or cold, how do I know if it was damaged?

You may not. Studies suggest that cold temperatures are generally tolerated. But even a few hours in extreme heat, such as inside a car in the summer, can degrade the medication. If the liquid in the clear window has become cloudy or brown, the injector needs to be replaced. Even so, exposure to extreme temperatures might compromise the injector without any obvious changes. If you suspect there was exposure to an extreme temperature, replace the injector.

How does the doctor decide on the dose of epinephrine for autoinjectors?

Most of the autoinjectors are sold with either 0.15 or 0.3 mg. The Auvi-Q has a 0.1-milligram dose, and the European Emerade has a 0.5-milligram dose. If epinephrine were dosed exactly, the recommendations are generally 0.01 milligrams per kilogram, up to 0.3 or 0.5 milligrams per dose. Manufacturers generally suggest the 0.1-milligram dose for infants weighing 16.5 to 33 pounds (7.5 to 15 kilograms), the 0.15-milligram dose for persons weighing between 33 and 66 pounds (15 to 30 kilograms), and the 0.3-milligram unit for persons at and above 66 pounds. Although these are recommended by the manufacturers, experts often recommend increasing doses at lower weight cutoffs to avoid significant underdosing. For example, a 65-pound child who received the 0.15-milligram dose is getting roughly half the suggested ideal dose. Table 4.3 shows the recommended weight ranges for epinephrine autoinjectors. Your doctor may suggest switching at slightly different weights depending on your specific history.

Table 4.3. Approximate Weight Ranges for Epinephrine Autoinjectors per Manufacturer Recommendations and Expert Recommendations

Dose in Autoinjector (milligrams)	Weight Range per Manufacturer	Weight Range (Approximate) per Expert Recommendations*
0.1	16.5 to 33 pounds (7.5 to 15 kilograms)	16.5 to less than 29 pounds (7.5 to less than 13 kilograms)
0.15	33 to 66 pounds (15 to 30 kilograms)	29 to 55 pounds (13 to less than 25 kilograms)
0.3	66 pounds and over (30 kilograms and over)	55 pounds and over (25 kilograms or more)

*Following these ranges avoids underdosing compared to generally accepted dosing. Switching points are approximate.

What can be done to give epinephrine to infants who are too small for the lowest autoinjector dose?

This is a difficult situation because the alternative to an autoinjector is to have a glass vial of epinephrine and a syringe. Studies suggest that using this means of treatment can be prone to errors. Experts currently recommend using the 0.1-milligram autoinjector for smaller infants, but this is currently only available from one manufacturer. If the 0.1-milligram injector is not available, experts also suggest using the 0.15-milligram autoinjector starting with infants who are 16.5 pounds (7.5 kilograms). Experts are also asking that manufacturers and regulatory agencies consider making more autoinjectors with a wider range of doses.

Does the injection hurt?

It feels like a pinch, but people often describe the relief they feel from symptoms rather than the pain from the injection.

Is giving the injection dangerous?

No, although it is possible to cause deep cuts in the skin if a child wiggles and moves while being injected. Read the autoinjector instructions carefully. Most autoinjectors release the medication quickly, and instructions generally suggest holding the device in place for shorter periods of time compared to prior years (for example, 3 seconds instead of 10). Additionally, take care to hold a child's leg still while injecting.

How can I overcome fear of self-injection?

If you think that you or your child would be reluctant to self-inject, you should discuss this openly with your physician. The safety of the medication should be emphasized, but some people have an aversion to needles that increases their reluctance to self-inject. Some allergists have advocated for having patients self-inject in the office, just to allay any fear about doing it during a reaction. Another approach is to use a sterile needle and syringe, under medical supervision, with no injection of medication, just to build confidence that the self-injection can be done. A 2017 study by Shemesh et al. suggested that this method is helpful for teenagers who are willing to try (see chapter 11).

What if I injected my finger with epinephrine by accident?

This is a common error when a person is attempting to give the treatment to another person. It underscores why it is essential to review how to use the injectors and to practice with trainers. If the thumb is accidentally injected, the blood vessels in the finger may spasm, reducing blood flow. This usually resolves by itself, but if your finger is discolored, you should go to an emergency room for treatment with a paste or injection that reverses the problem. Also, don't forget to use another injector to administer the epinephrine to the person who needs it.

What can you tell me to encourage me/my child to use the epinephrine?

Injected epinephrine is a very good treatment for asthma and was used routinely to treat wheeze prior to the widespread use of asthma inhalers. It was routine to get these injections for a simple wheeze. Some people now think it is dramatic to have this injection, but it was not a big deal decades ago. Here are some important observations to consider:

Giving the epinephrine promptly . . .
• reduces the chance of a bad outcome, including fatality
• reduces the chance of needing more than one dose
• reduces the chance of being hospitalized
• makes you feel better quickly

Antihistamines

What does an antihistamine do?

Antihistamines block the histamine that is released from allergy cells during an allergic reaction. Histamine is partly responsible for the itching, redness, and swelling during an allergic reaction. Many powerful chemicals are released during anaphylaxis, however, and an antihistamine cannot treat anaphylaxis.

If antihistamines cannot treat anaphylaxis, why do symptoms sometimes get better with antihistamines alone?

Allergic reactions may improve on their own, or the symptoms may be mild enough to respond to the antihistamines.

What antihistamines are available?

There are many over-the-counter antihistamines, as well as a few prescription types. They can be sold under brand names or generic names. The "side," or inactive, ingredients may differ among the formulations and between the brands and the generics. Examples of popular over-the-counter antihistamines include diphenhydramine (Benadryl), cetirizine (Zyrtec), and fexofenadine (Allegra). There are various formulations (capsules, liquid, meltaways, melting strips, tablets, and so on). All antihistamines have generally the same actions, reducing itching and swelling. Their onset of action, length of action, and degree of sedation (sleepiness) can differ. The two forms used most often for food-allergic reactions are diphenhydramine and cetirizine. Watch out for combination forms (for example, those with decongestant or pain medications in the same formulation) that are sold to treat various cold and flu symptoms. For an allergic reaction, you want to purchase the basic types that have one active ingredient.

How long does it take for an antihistamine to work?

About 30 minutes for diphenhydramine and cetirizine. When symptoms appear to improve promptly after taking an antihistamine, this usually means the symptoms would have improved on their own without treatment.

Does it matter what form of antihistamine is taken (dissolvable, liquid, pill, or other form)?

For additional treatment during anaphylaxis, use a form that can be absorbed as quickly as possible. Thus all forms *except* capsules and pills might be preferentially used. Often, convenience is an issue because the antihistamines are carried along with epinephrine in a "kit" or pack. Some people prefer to carry dissolvable forms or premeasured foil pouches. You should explore options and practice opening the different forms to see what works best for you.

How are antihistamines dosed?

The dosing of diphenhydramine is generally 12.5 milligrams for every 22 pounds, up to about 50 milligrams. The dosing for cetirizine is generally 2.5 milligrams for ages 2 through 5 and 5 to 10 milligrams for ages 6 and older. Your doctor may suggest slightly different dosing for use during an allergic reaction, usually going toward the higher ranges for weight or age.

Should antihistamines be part of a treatment plan for anaphylaxis?
Antihistamines are generally part of an anaphylaxis treatment plan to provide additional comfort care.

What are the side effects of antihistamines?
Most forms cause sedation, but the degree of sedation can differ. For example, diphenhydramine is more sedating, in general, than cetirizine. Some people experience the opposite effect, feeling restless.

In anaphylaxis, what should be given first, epinephrine or an antihistamine?
If anaphylaxis is occurring, the priority is to give epinephrine.

If symptoms are not getting better after a dose of antihistamines, can more be given?
Many physicians suggest taking a bit more antihistamine, but it can take 30 minutes for the dose to take effect. The types of symptoms must be considered as well. Any progressive symptoms or severe symptoms, as described in the previous sections, should be treated with epinephrine, without waiting for or expecting the antihistamine to treat these symptoms.

If a person is already taking antihistamines for a condition like hay fever, and they have a food-allergic reaction, can more antihistamines be taken?
Yes, this is a reasonable approach.

Can being on an antihistamine for hay fever or another allergic problem reduce early and mild symptoms after a food allergen is eaten?
Yes. For example, it may reduce mouth itch or some hives. It would not necessarily affect progression of a reaction to anaphylaxis. Again, antihistamines do not treat anaphylaxis!

Is it dangerous or problematic to be on an antihistamine continuously if you have a severe food allergy?
There is a hypothetical concern that being on an antihistamine might reduce the milder initial symptoms of an allergic reaction, resulting in the person continuing to eat a food with an allergen and perhaps getting a larger dose of the food. But allergists advocate appropriate treatment of

allergic conditions with antihistamines regardless of there being a potentially severe food allergy. There is no reason to suffer with hay fever or itchy skin rashes because of a theoretical concern about using antihistamines with a severe food allergy. Additionally, to maintain safety, it is not appropriate to depend on experiencing initial mild symptoms from a meal (which often does not occur even off antihistamines). One should be careful to obtain safe foods through label reading and good communication. Whether or not mild initial symptoms occur, however, epinephrine, not antihistamines, is the necessary treatment for anaphylaxis.

Additional Medications and Treatments for Anaphylaxis

What additional treatments are given to people having anaphylaxis?
In addition to epinephrine and antihistamines, asthma medications may be given for those with asthma and wheezing. An emergency room or ambulance has the option to administer various additional treatments, such as oxygen, intravenous fluids, medications to support breathing and blood pressure, and steroids. The emergency room also has access to machines that support breathing, if needed.

What type of asthma medications might be given during anaphylaxis?
A bronchodilator, the asthma "rescue" medication that is prescribed to relieve wheezing from asthma, may be given.

Can a bronchodilator be given for wheezing during anaphylaxis?
It can be given as an *additional* treatment to epinephrine, but it CANNOT be depended on to treat anaphylaxis on its own. Epinephrine is an excellent treatment for wheezing and was a treatment for asthma prior to the invention of asthma inhalers.

Can a bronchodilator be given in place of epinephrine for anaphylaxis?
Never.

What are steroids?
Corticosteroids are an anti-inflammatory medication that is often given to

reduce wheezing in severe asthma exacerbations. These are different from the type of steroids abused to build muscle.

When are steroids given for anaphylaxis?
Many physicians will give steroids when there has been a severe allergic reaction. The benefit of this therapy is unclear.

Why are steroids given for anaphylaxis?
It is presumed that the steroid will quell later swelling in the lungs, as they do for asthma exacerbations, and perhaps assist in reducing swelling elsewhere. This remains unproven, however. A 2020 expert guideline concluded that this treatment does not prevent reemergence of anaphylaxis symptoms.

How long does it take for a steroid to treat symptoms?
Approximately four to six hours, which underscores why steroids are not part of an immediate emergency plan to treat anaphylaxis, as epinephrine is.

Can steroids replace epinephrine to treat anaphylaxis?
Never.

Should I carry steroids to treat anaphylaxis?
Generally, no. They cannot improve symptoms of anaphylaxis and may deter proper therapy. Sometimes physicians prescribe them to carry if a person is going to travel to remote areas, hours away from any medical attention, presumably to assist with the later-onset asthma symptoms of anaphylaxis that sometimes occurs, or to assist in treating a severe asthma exacerbation.

How long should steroids be continued after they are given for anaphylaxis?
Some physicians prescribe them for several days, similar to what is done for an asthma exacerbation, but this approach has not been studied. If there are no further symptoms, there is no reason to continue steroids.

What is Singulair (montelukast), and can it be used to treat anaphylaxis?
Singulair is an oral medication used for asthma and hay fever. It blocks one of the inflammatory pathways that is important in allergy, but it has not

been studied for treatment of anaphylaxis. It is NOT recommended as a treatment during anaphylaxis.

When waiting for help, how should people undergoing anaphylaxis be treated?

They should be kept calm and be positioned comfortably. This may be a sitting position for a person having trouble breathing. In severe anaphylaxis, particularly if symptoms suggest poor blood circulation, the person should lie down. If the person is vomiting, however, lying on one side is safer, to prevent choking.

Why is it suggested to lie down for severe anaphylaxis?

When blood circulation is poor, gravity can pull blood away from important areas of the body, such as the brain and internal organs. Lying allows gravity to help get blood where it is needed. Once people with severe anaphylaxis are lying down, they should be kept in this position until they are stabilized by medical experts; there may be danger in standing them up.

Why is it possibly dangerous for a person who is having severe anaphylaxis to stand?

If a person has severe anaphylaxis with low blood pressure (anaphylactic shock) and is not fully treated, standing up might suddenly pool blood into the legs, leaving the heart with nothing to pump, which could be fatal. This has rarely occurred in adults.

Does charcoal provide any relief for anaphylaxis?

Activated charcoal (not the kind used in a barbeque) is a medicinal treatment used for poisonings. It has been theorized as a treatment for food anaphylaxis, to absorb the allergen from the gut, but this has not been studied adequately. Although some emergency room physicians may consider this treatment, drawbacks include potential lung damage if the charcoal is vomited and accidentally inhaled.

Written Emergency Plans, Education, Medical Identification Jewelry, and Management Issues

What is a written emergency plan for anaphylaxis?

These brief written plans, sometimes called anaphylaxis action plans, allergy and anaphylaxis emergency plans, and so forth, describe the actions to be taken in the event of an allergic reaction such as anaphylaxis. They are generally created for caregivers of children in schools or camps, but they are helpful for all caregivers and for food-allergic adults as well.

What are the key components of a written food anaphylaxis plan?

The plan identifies the allergic individual (often with a picture), the person's allergies, whether he or she has asthma (a risk for more severe reactions), the typical symptoms to watch for, what treatments to provide if those symptoms occur, and contact information. Many plans include additional instructions about the treatments.

Who writes the emergency plan for food allergy?

A physician or a physician's qualified assistant.

Where can I find a written food allergy emergency action plan?

If your doctor or school does not have their own, you can download one from a variety of websites. Figure 4.1 shows the plan from the American Academy of Pediatrics, and figure 4.2 shows the plan from Food Allergy Research & Education.

What is medical identification jewelry?

This is a bracelet or pendant that has a medical insignia and describes the medical condition and potential severe risks, for example, food allergy and anaphylaxis.

Why is medical identification jewelry recommended?

In the event the victim becomes incapacitated during a reaction, medical identification jewelry can inform passersby and medical professionals. For children, this may also be a helpful reminder to others about not offering unsafe foods.

Where do I get medical identification jewelry?

Several companies make them. The largest one is a not-for-profit foundation, MedicAlert (www.medicalert.org). You may want to list some of your food allergies and indicate "anaphylaxis" or "food allergy and anaphylaxis." This foundation also has an option to keep your personal medical information on file so that a responder can get additional details by contacting MedicAlert.

What are additional ways to have notification about allergies?

The cell phone has become a fixture for most people. Having allergy notification there can be an additional help. You can use ICE.

How do you get a cell phone to show emergency information, and what is ICE?

ICE stands for "In Case of Emergency." Various cell phone apps allow your cell phone or smartphone to call emergency services, present medical information, and alert responders about medical problems, including food allergies, often through a health-related app. Cell phone service providers may also offer an ICE icon. At minimum, an emergency contact can be created using ICE ahead of the name (for example, by typing "ICE" and then the name of the contact), and the specific medical problems such as allergies can be added in the notes field.

What other aspects of medical care should a person at risk for food anaphylaxis address?

Keeping asthma under good control.

Why is it important to keep asthma in good control for people at risk of food anaphylaxis?

It is presumed that a vulnerable lung increases the risk of having breathing problems during anaphylaxis. Although having stable, well-controlled asthma is still a risk factor, it is more dangerous to have anaphylaxis when the lung is already wheezing and swelling.

Allergy and Anaphylaxis Emergency Plan

American Academy of Pediatrics
DEDICATED TO THE HEALTH OF ALL CHILDREN®

Child's name: _____ Date of plan: _____

Date of birth: ____/____/_____ Age _____ Weight: _____kg

Child has allergy to _____

Attach
child's
photo

Child has asthma.   ☐ Yes ☐ No (If yes, higher chance severe reaction)
Child has had anaphylaxis.   ☐ Yes ☐ No
Child may carry medicine.   ☐ Yes ☐ No
Child may give him/herself medicine. ☐ Yes ☐ No (If child refuses/is unable to self-treat, an adult must give medicine)

IMPORTANT REMINDER
Anaphylaxis is a potentially life-threating, severe allergic reaction. If in doubt, give epinephrine.

For Severe Allergy and Anaphylaxis **What to look for**	**Give epinephrine!** **What to do**

If child has ANY of these severe symptoms after eating the food or having a sting, **give epinephrine**.
• Shortness of breath, wheezing, or coughing
• Skin color is pale or has a bluish color
• Weak pulse
• Fainting or dizziness
• Tight or hoarse throat
• Trouble breathing or swallowing
• Swelling of lips or tongue that bother breathing
• Vomiting or diarrhea (if severe or combined with other symptoms)
• Many hives or redness over body
• Feeling of "doom," confusion, altered consciousness, or agitation
 	
☐ **SPECIAL SITUATION**: If this box is checked, child has an extremely severe allergy to an insect sting or the following food(s): _____. Even if child has MILD symptoms after a sting or eating these foods, **give epinephrine**.
	1. Inject epinephrine right away! Note time when epinephrine was given.
	2. Call 911.
	   • Ask for ambulance with epinephrine.
	   • Tell rescue squad when epinephrine was given.
	3. Stay with child and:
	   • Call parents and child's doctor.
	   • Give a second dose of epinephrine, if symptoms get worse, continue, or do not get better in 5 minutes.
	   • Keep child lying on back. If the child vomits or has trouble breathing, keep child lying on his or her side.
	4. Give other medicine, if prescribed. Do not use other medicine in place of epinephrine.
	   • Antihistamine
	   • Inhaler/bronchodilator

For Mild Allergic Reaction **What to look for**	**Monitor child** **What to do**
If child has had any mild symptoms, **monitor child.** Symptoms may include: • Itchy nose, sneezing, itchy mouth • A few hives • Mild stomach nausea or discomfort	Stay with child and: • Watch child closely. • Give antihistamine (if prescribed). • Call parents and child's doctor. • If more than 1 symptom or symptoms of severe allergy/anaphylaxis develop, use epinephrine. (See "For Severe Allergy and Anaphylaxis.")

Medicines/Doses
Epinephrine, intramuscular (list type): _____ Dose:☐ 0.10 mg (7.5 kg to less than13 kg)*
                                                                              ☐ 0.15 mg (13 kg to less than 25 kg)
                                                                              ☐ 0.30 mg (25 kg or more)
Antihistamine, by mouth (type and dose): _____ (*Use 0.15 mg, if 0.10 mg is not available)
Other (for example, inhaler/bronchodilator if child has asthma): _____

_____ _____ _____ _____
Parent/Guardian Authorization Signature   **Date**   **Physician/HCP Authorization Signature**   **Date**

Figure 4.1. American Academy of Pediatrics' Allergy and Anaphylaxis Emergency Plan. Reproduced with permission from *Pediatrics*, Vol. 139, © 2017 by the AAP.

Allergy and Anaphylaxis Emergency Plan

American Academy of Pediatrics
DEDICATED TO THE HEALTH OF ALL CHILDREN®

Child's name: _____ Date of plan: _____

Additional Instructions:

Contacts

Call 911 / Rescue squad: _____

Doctor: _____ Phone: _____

Parent/Guardian: _____ Phone: _____

Parent/Guardian: _____ Phone: _____

Other Emergency Contacts

Name/Relationship: _____ Phone: _____

Name/Relationship: _____ Phone: _____

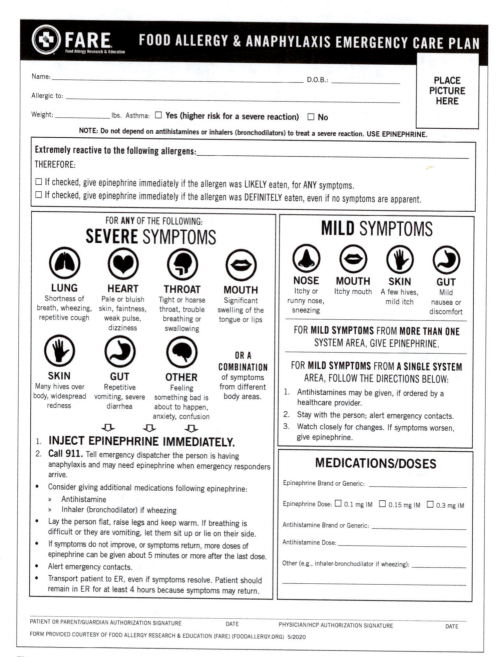

Figure 4.2. Food Allergy Research & Education's Food Allergy and Anaphylaxis Emergency Care Plan. © 2019 FARE. Used with permission.

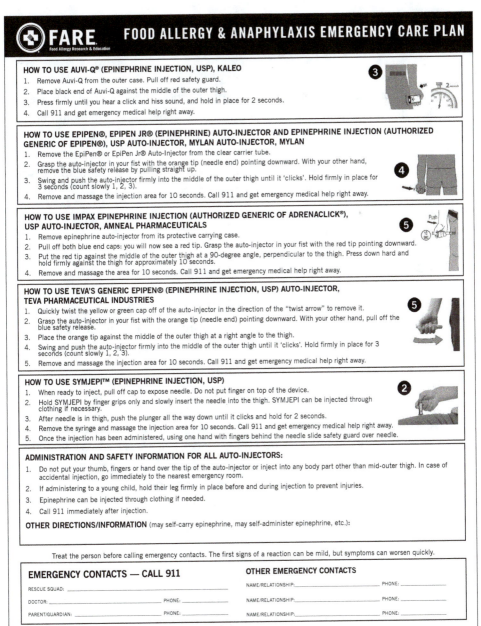

FOOD ALLERGY & ANAPHYLAXIS EMERGENCY CARE PLAN

FARE — Food Allergy Research & Education

HOW TO USE AUVI-Q® (EPINEPHRINE INJECTION, USP), KALEO
1. Remove Auvi-Q from the outer case. Pull off red safety guard.
2. Place black end of Auvi-Q against the middle of the outer thigh.
3. Press firmly until you hear a click and hiss sound, and hold in place for 2 seconds.
4. Call 911 and get emergency medical help right away.

HOW TO USE EPIPEN®, EPIPEN JR® (EPINEPHRINE) AUTO-INJECTOR AND EPINEPHRINE INJECTION (AUTHORIZED GENERIC OF EPIPEN®), USP AUTO-INJECTOR, MYLAN AUTO-INJECTOR, MYLAN
1. Remove the EpiPen® or EpiPen Jr® Auto-Injector from the clear carrier tube.
2. Grasp the auto-injector in your fist with the orange tip (needle end) pointing downward. With your other hand, remove the blue safety release by pulling straight up.
3. Swing and push the auto-injector firmly into the middle of the outer thigh until it 'clicks'. Hold firmly in place for 3 seconds (count slowly 1, 2, 3).
4. Remove and massage the injection area for 10 seconds. Call 911 and get emergency medical help right away.

HOW TO USE IMPAX EPINEPHRINE INJECTION (AUTHORIZED GENERIC OF ADRENACLICK®), USP AUTO-INJECTOR, AMNEAL PHARMACEUTICALS
1. Remove epinephrine auto-injector from its protective carrying case.
2. Pull off both blue end caps: you will now see a red tip. Grasp the auto-injector in your fist with the red tip pointing downward.
3. Put the red tip against the middle of the outer thigh at a 90-degree angle, perpendicular to the thigh. Press down hard and hold firmly against the thigh for approximately 10 seconds.
4. Remove and massage the area for 10 seconds. Call 911 and get emergency medical help right away.

HOW TO USE TEVA'S GENERIC EPIPEN® (EPINEPHRINE INJECTION, USP) AUTO-INJECTOR, TEVA PHARMACEUTICAL INDUSTRIES
1. Quickly twist the yellow or green cap off of the auto-injector in the direction of the "twist arrow" to remove it.
2. Grasp the auto-injector in your fist with the orange tip (needle end) pointing downward. With your other hand, pull off the blue safety release.
3. Place the orange tip against the middle of the outer thigh at a right angle to the thigh.
4. Swing and push the auto-injector firmly into the middle of the outer thigh until it 'clicks'. Hold firmly in place for 3 seconds (count slowly 1, 2, 3).
5. Remove and massage the injection area for 10 seconds. Call 911 and get emergency medical help right away.

HOW TO USE SYMJEPI™ (EPINEPHRINE INJECTION, USP)
1. When ready to inject, pull off cap to expose needle. Do not put finger on top of the device.
2. Hold SYMJEPI by finger grips only and slowly insert the needle into the thigh. SYMJEPI can be injected through clothing if necessary.
3. After needle is in thigh, push the plunger all the way down until it clicks and hold for 2 seconds.
4. Remove the syringe and massage the injection area for 10 seconds. Call 911 and get emergency medical help right away.
5. Once the injection has been administered, using one hand with fingers behind the needle slide safety guard over needle.

ADMINISTRATION AND SAFETY INFORMATION FOR ALL AUTO-INJECTORS:
1. Do not put your thumb, fingers or hand over the tip of the auto-injector or inject into any body part other than mid-outer thigh. In case of accidental injection, go immediately to the nearest emergency room.
2. If administering to a young child, hold their leg firmly in place before and during injection to prevent injuries.
3. Epinephrine can be injected through clothing if needed.
4. Call 911 immediately after injection.

OTHER DIRECTIONS/INFORMATION (may self-carry epinephrine, may self-administer epinephrine, etc.):

Treat the person before calling emergency contacts. The first signs of a reaction can be mild, but symptoms can worsen quickly.

EMERGENCY CONTACTS — CALL 911
RESCUE SQUAD: _____

DOCTOR: _____ PHONE: _____

PARENT/GUARDIAN: _____ PHONE: _____

OTHER EMERGENCY CONTACTS
NAME/RELATIONSHIP:_____ PHONE: _____

NAME/RELATIONSHIP:_____ PHONE: _____

NAME/RELATIONSHIP:_____ PHONE: _____

FORM PROVIDED COURTESY OF FOOD ALLERGY RESEARCH & EDUCATION (FARE) (FOODALLERGY.ORG) 5/2020

Chapter Lessons

Here are six brief cases of allergic reactions followed by multiple-choice options for actions that could be taken. Think about what you would do, and check your answers against the ones I provide at the end.

Case 1. A child with a peanut allergy ate a peanut a minute ago and now has three hives on her face and no other symptoms:

- (a) Inject epinephrine and give antihistamine
- (b) Give antihistamine and watch

Case 2. Your 16-year-old sitter calls to say that your 3-year-old child, who is severely allergic to eggs, milk, and peanuts and has had severe reactions in the past, may have eaten something he is allergic to because he has hives on his face. The sitter does not think he is coughing or having any other problems, but he stopped playing with his ball. What should you tell her to do?

- (a) Inject epinephrine and give antihistamine
- (b) Give antihistamine and watch

Case 3. You are in a bakery with your 18-month-old in your arms. She is allergic to peanuts. While you are eyeing a cake, she grabs a cookie, which you know because you hear chewing and see crumbs spilling from her full mouth. You jostle her and in a panic scream, "How did you grab that?" She immediately stops breathing and is turning blue.

- (a) Inject epinephrine and give antihistamine
- (b) Give antihistamine and watch
- (c) Do something else

Case 4. Your child, who has egg and milk allergies, ate a safe lunch. He also has asthma and has been developing a cold. He went to play outside and came back inside with a hacking cough and wheezing. He has no other symptoms.

- (a) Inject epinephrine and give antihistamine
- (b) Give antihistamine and watch
- (c) Give an asthma inhaler (bronchodilator)

Case 5. A child with severe egg allergy is finger painting. She develops an itchy eye that swells shut while she is rubbing it. There are no other symptoms. The teacher realizes that she had smoothed the paint with egg white.

(a) Inject epinephrine and give antihistamine

(b) Give antihistamine and watch

Case 6. A 19-year-old has a severe peanut allergy. She is carrying her self-injectable epinephrine. Her friend opens a bag of potato chips, and, after eating a few, she asks if it is okay that they are flavored with peanut oil and that she is eating them in the same room. The girl with peanut allergy says that she feels like she is having trouble breathing. She looks pale. She says her fingers feel numb and she might vomit.

(a) Inject epinephrine and take antihistamine

(b) Take antihistamine and watch

(c) Do something else

Answers to Case Studies

1: (a) or (b). Either choice could be correct. It would likely depend on knowing more about the child. If the child has had extremely severe past reactions to peanuts, with breathing problems, for example, one might go ahead and use the epinephrine. If past reactions were all mild skin rashes, it would be reasonable to give antihistamines and watch carefully.

2: (a). I would suggest giving the epinephrine. In this case, it is a concern that an inexperienced person is making the decisions. The child already has hives, is behaving differently, and the 16-year-old may not be able to monitor the reaction appropriately. The child is also known to have multiple severe allergies and apparently ate something that was an allergen. I think the best decision is to have the sitter inject epinephrine and call 911.

3: (c). You may have chosen to inject epinephrine because there is a breathing problem. This is a bit of a trick question, however. An allergic reaction should not result in an inability to breathe seconds after eating the allergen. That would just be too fast for an allergic reaction. Here, the baby had a mouth full of cookie and was jostled. Most likely, she is choking and needs a Heimlich maneuver to dislodge the cookie from her windpipe.

4: (c). Although wheezing and coughing suggest the need to treat a food-allergic reaction with epinephrine, this child has asthma and has two reasons to wheeze: his respiratory infection and exercise. He also ate a safe lunch, so there is no suggestion that he ate a food to which he is allergic. Therefore giving an asthma inhaler is the best choice. If you did give this child epinephrine, it would also help his wheezing.

5: (b) It is most reasonable to give antihistamines and watch. There is no evidence that the girl ate the egg-laden paint, but she did rub it in her eye. The eye is sensitive and swells easily. For example, people with pollen allergy may experience significant eyelid swelling just from pollen in the air. It is not likely that a skin or an eye exposure will progress to anaphylaxis.

6: (a) or (b) or (c). The girl is describing problems affecting her gut, breathing, and possibly circulation. These would normally suggest anaphylaxis, and it is prudent to respond by giving epinephrine, but it is probably unnecessary in this case. Her symptoms also match those of anxiety and hyperventilation (breathing fast, hard, and heavy). It is most likely that the girl is nervous about being near the peanut oil and is having a panic attack. This response is common because people react with anxiety to something they know can hurt them. Imagine having a gun pointed at your head. You might breathe heavily and faint, but that is not an allergy.

Hyperventilating causes imbalances in blood acids that result in feeling light-headed and in tingling or numbness in the fingers. She might benefit from being calmed and breathing into a bag (choice [c]); however, given the uncertainty in the moment, it may be reasonable to inject epinephrine and sort out the circumstances later. In this case, not injecting epinephrine is also reasonable because there are many reasons to suspect there is no allergic reaction: anaphylaxis is not likely from air exposure, peanut oil often has no proteins from peanut, and even if the oil had peanut protein, it would not permeate the air. The final decision would probably depend on the confidence of an observer, but if the girl was the person deciding to inject, I would suggest that she go ahead and do so.

CHAPTER 5

Chronic Health Problems Caused by Food Allergy

This chapter provides answers to questions about several chronic illnesses that are caused by food allergy. I describe how chronic allergic symptoms may be related to foods, and I discuss medical conditions that are not so clearly related to food allergies.

General Questions about Chronic Illnesses and Foods

Can food allergies cause symptoms that are persistent (chronic) rather than sudden after a food is eaten?
Yes. Many chronic skin and gastrointestinal illnesses are associated with food allergies.

What chronic allergic illnesses can be related to food allergies?
Food allergy can contribute to atopic dermatitis and various gastrointestinal illnesses in infants, children, and adults.

Respiratory Symptoms

Is asthma caused by food allergies?
Generally not. Triggers of asthma include respiratory infections, exercise, and allergens in the air, such as pollens, dust mites, and animal danders. During a severe allergic reaction to food, asthma may flare. Studies suggest

that it is uncommon for ingestion of a food to lead to the chronic lung inflammation that causes asthma. For some people with chronic asthma, however, food allergy does play a role.

How often does food allergy contribute to chronic asthma?

Various studies of people with asthma show that foods contribute to asthma episodes in fewer than 1 in 25 asthmatic children and even less frequently among adults. Even so, isolated chronic asthma—without food allergy, skin reactions, or gut symptoms—is rare.

How can I tell if my asthma is caused by food allergies?

The first assumption should be that they are not related. If there is a strong suspicion, however, and the asthma is not responding well to medical treatments, testing can be done. If testing is positive, it would likely require a trial period of avoiding the suspected food and then reintroducing it, under medical supervision, to determine whether there is a relationship.

Is hay fever caused by food allergies?

Generally not. Nasal symptoms—itching, sneezing, runny nose, and congestion—are common during a food-allergic reaction, but chronic hay fever is typically attributable to allergens in the air, such as pollens.

Hives and Swelling

Are chronic hives, those occurring almost daily for many weeks, caused by food allergies?

Usually not. A few studies suggest that the chemical nature of food additives may contribute to chronic hives in fewer than 5% of cases. As a chemical effect, this is not an allergy. True food allergies are rarely related to chronic hives.

Why would food allergy not be a likely cause of chronic hives?

Hives are the most common symptom of an allergic reaction to food, but they typically occur in minutes and fade within an hour of eating the causal food. They do not recur unless the food is eaten again. People with an illness called "chronic urticaria," or chronic hives, have the rash on most days for longer than six weeks. It would be quite odd for a person to eat the causal food, experience hives, and then eat the food again and again without realizing a connection.

What is the cause of chronic urticaria?

When someone has hives, sometimes also with swelling (edema) of the face, lips, or other areas of the body, for a week or two, the most common trigger is a viral infection. If the hives and swellings are unrelenting for many weeks, they are most often due to a type of autoimmune response, when the body is attacking its own allergy cells. People with chronic hives have a higher rate of making antibodies against molecules on their allergy cells, hence activating them to cause hives. These individuals are also at risk of developing other illnesses where the body is attacking itself, for example, thyroid problems.

Is food ever a contributing factor to chronic hives?

There are theories that some components of foods might cause or contribute to chronic hives. A few studies suggest that chemicals in foods might cause hives in some people. Because the theory is not about an allergic reaction, the term "pseudoallergen" has been used.

What are pseudoallergens?

According to this theory, food additives, vasoactive substances such as histamine, and some natural substances in fruits, vegetables, and spices contribute to chronic hives. A trial of a pseudoallergen-free diet is recommended by proponents of this theory.

What is involved with a pseudoallergen-free diet?

The list of foods to avoid is extensive. One group suggests avoiding the following: additives such as E100–E1518; alcohol; antioxidants; baking agents; biscuits; breads with additional grains, herbs, or other such added ingredients; cakes; candy, chewing gum, and similar products; dried fruits and fruit juices; eggs and pasta made with eggs; emulsifiers; flavoring agents, foaming agents, potentiators, and stabilizers; gelling agents; herbal teas; humectants; margarine and mayonnaise; potato chips; preservatives and artificial colors; modified starches; seafood; separating agents; sesame; smoked meats; spices and herbs (except salt and chives); sweeteners; thickening matter; and certain vegetables, including artichokes, mushrooms, olives, peas, rhubarb, spinach, sweet peppers, and tomatoes. The diet allows only fresh foods—no preserved foods—except deep-frozen foods without any additives.

How long is the pseudoallergen-free diet for chronic hives to be tried?
Three weeks.

What is the success rate of the pseudoallergen-free diet for chronic hives?
One group claims a success rate of one in six, with up to one in three having some improvement.

Is a pseudoallergen-free diet for chronic hives recommended?
There are only a few small studies and no large studies comparing people who tried the diet to those who did not. Some researchers claim that the diet might cure the hives because, after many months, the foods could be added back without recurrence of hives. I am suspicious that, without a comparison group treated with a placebo diet, the effect of this extensive diet is unproven. Some of the people eating a pseudoallergen-free diet would likely have resolved their hives after weeks or months regardless of whether they followed the diet. The diet is healthful, though, so I would not deter a person from trying it. It should be done in coordination with a physician, and after discussing the nature of the illness, standard treatments, and consideration of alternative causes of chronic hives (and associated illnesses, as discussed above).

What is pressure-related swelling?
There is a rare condition where pressure on the skin results in hives (urticaria) or swelling (angioedema) several hours later. There is an even more uncommon condition where this occurs only if the person eats a specific food.

Atopic Dermatitis (Eczema)

What is atopic dermatitis?
Atopic dermatitis, more generally called eczema, is a skin condition. The main symptom is an itchy rash that tends to run in families; it occurs in people with other allergic problems, such as asthma, and it follows a pat-

tern on the skin that varies by age. For infants, the scalp, face, chest, arms, and legs are often affected. Children and adults tend to have the rashes in the folds of the knees, elbows, and neck, along with other areas. Figure 5.1 shows common areas affected by atopic dermatitis.

What causes atopic dermatitis?
Many different triggers inflame the hyperirritable skin of someone with eczema. The skin is also prone to infection and has a defective barrier, so it dries out easily.

Is eczema caused by food allergies?
There is some controversy about whether foods can contribute to the chronic rashes of atopic dermatitis. About one in three children with more than mild atopic dermatitis have food allergies, including anaphylaxis. Because there are many other triggers, the extent to which eczema in children is primarily due to food allergy is unclear. Some children (and much less frequently adults) do clearly have food-related flaring of their atopic dermatitis.

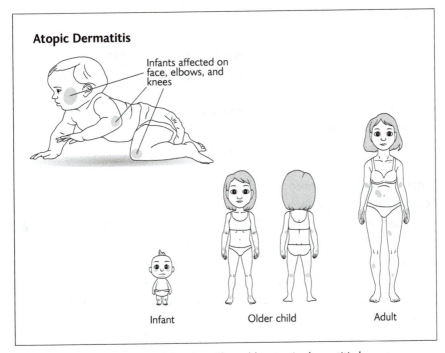

Figure 5.1. Common areas of the skin affected by atopic dermatitis by age.

What triggers eczema/atopic dermatitis other than food?

The primary triggers are irritants, such as sweating, dryness, soaps, scratching, clothing that holds in moisture or is itchy like wool, infections, stress, and allergens from the environment, such as animal dander and pollen.

How is atopic dermatitis treated?

Treatment may require hydrating baths (long soaks in lukewarm water); application of topical medications that reduce inflammation, such as steroids and other anti-inflammatory creams or ointments; antibiotics to reduce infection; and moisturizers and creams to improve the skin barrier. Irritants are reduced by using mild soaps or by double-rinsing clothes and choosing cotton rather than wool or polyester clothing. Keeping fingernails short will reduce the damage from scratching. Antihistamines may be used to lessen itching and to induce sedation at bedtime, which further minimizes scratching.

How is food allergy related to eczema/atopic dermatitis?

Some studies show that removal of a particular food allergen can help relieve symptoms and that the symptoms increase when the food is returned to the diet (unless the allergies are outgrown).

Which foods may contribute to eczema/atopic dermatitis?

The most likely triggers for children are eggs, milk, wheat, and soy.

What are the benefits of identifying and removing foods to treat eczema/atopic dermatitis?

There may be improved control of the rash.

What are the risks of removing foods that may contribute to eczema/atopic dermatitis?

There are several, as shown in table 5.1. Removing a food that is a stable part of the diet but that tests positively as an allergen rarely results in the allergy being more immediate and severe when the food is reintroduced. Although this is an uncommon occurrence, it is the reason medical treatments should be tried and maximized prior to removing foods. This is discussed further in chapter 3.

Table 5.1. Risk and Benefit of Removing a Food from the Diet to Treat Atopic Dermatitis

Possible Benefit	Possible Risk
Improved rash	Nutritional deficits
Reduced itching	Social issues owing to avoidance (restriction of foods at social activities)
Less medication	New or more severe allergies to the foods removed from the diet

Who with atopic dermatitis should be tested for food allergies?

Experts have suggested that food allergies should be considered for people with atopic dermatitis who have noticed allergic reactions to foods or flaring of their eczema rash with foods. Another group that may warrant an investigation for food allergy are children under age 5 who have more than mild atopic dermatitis and whose rash is not responding well to standard treatments. A good skin care treatment regimen should be tried before considering food allergies, however, because removal of foods from the diet carries the risks mentioned above.

How does one identify what foods may contribute to atopic dermatitis?

Assuming the eczema rash did not respond well to medical treatments, foods can be considered as possible triggers. Typically, tests are performed to identify possible triggers, focusing on the few foods that are most often the cause. The suspected food is removed for a few weeks and returned to the diet under medical supervision. See chapter 3 for more details about diagnosis.

How easy is it to determine which foods might be contributing to atopic dermatitis?

It is extremely difficult. In studies of children with atopic dermatitis, most of the foods the family and patient suspected to be triggering the rash were disproven as triggers.

Why is it difficult to determine which foods contribute to atopic dermatitis?

There are two reasons. First, atopic dermatitis has a naturally waxing and waning course, which can be misleading when trying to make causal connections to foods. To make matters worse, some studies suggest that the symptoms can arise in the day or two after the food is eaten. This means that if you add a food, any flaring of the eczema in the next day or two could be attributed to the food when in reality the rash might have naturally flared.

The second hurdle is that atopic dermatitis improves from medical management but is not cured. This means that a few days of skin care may significantly improve the rash, only to have it flare up when treatments are withdrawn. Often, there is reluctance to treat with medications, and treatments are stopped when the rash improves. This approach is often doomed to fail because the medication is stopped and the trialed food is started at the same time. This can lead to the false impression that the food caused the flare when really the lack of continued medical treatment was the reason. Trials of adding foods to the diet should be undertaken during consistent treatment and when the skin is in good repair.

What is the suggested approach to determine whether foods are contributing to eczema?

The fundamental diagnostic tests described in chapter 3 (medical history, skin tests, blood tests, oral food challenges) should be administered. It is important not to change the daily treatment regimen while trials of food elimination and oral food challenge are undertaken. If the skin responds extremely well to medical therapy, it is beneficial to work with your doctor to attain the best management with the least amount of medication, perhaps in lieu of removing foods if this is achievable. Recall that atopic dermatitis is a skin disorder and that there are many triggers. If management with skin treatments is failing and a food is the cause, however, removal from the diet can be helpful.

What is a "fixed food eruption"?

This is an uncommon problem where an eczema-like rash develops in the same spot on the skin and lasts for days after a specific food is eaten.

Gastrointestinal and Digestive Illnesses

What stomach, digestive, or intestinal symptoms are triggered by foods?
The gut experiences only a few symptoms: pain, heartburn (acid reflux), nausea, vomiting, diarrhea, and poor nutrient absorption, leading to weight loss, poor weight gain, or growth failure. Foods can cause these symptoms either because of an allergy or for other reasons. Most gut problems, however, are not due to a food allergy.

Can chronic gut symptoms be attributed to foods?
Unlike most symptoms of a food allergy, where symptoms happen soon after a food is eaten and resolve fairly quickly afterward, chronic gut symptoms are not so clearly related to particular meals. For example, a person may be experiencing symptoms such as frequent pain, vomiting, and diarrhea that do not simply follow specific meals.

What kinds of symptoms are likely when foods are causing chronic allergic gut symptoms?
The most common symptoms include stomach pain, pain with swallowing, nausea, vomiting, diarrhea (especially with blood), heartburn/reflux, and poor weight gain or growth.

When should gut symptoms alert a person that there is a food allergy?
There are two ways that gut symptoms might be caused by a food allergy: (1) when symptoms of pain, nausea, vomiting, or diarrhea occur soon after a meal and (2) when symptoms have characteristics often seen in food allergies that affect the gut. These symptoms are consistent with a diagnosis of medical disorders called proctocolitis, enterocolitis, and eosinophilic gut disease.

Colic, Constipation, and Reflux

What is infant colic?
Colic is defined by frequent long periods of inconsolable crying. The strict medical definition of colic requires that an otherwise healthy infant show

unexplained fussing or crying for over three hours a day, more than three days a week, for longer than three weeks. Most parents, however, would consider their infant to be "colicky" with much less intense or extended periods of crying. Remember, too, that there may be medical reasons for inconsolable crying, anything from severe gut disease to having a hair wrapped tightly around a finger or toe, so always discuss this with your doctor.

Is infant colic due to food allergy?

Although some studies have linked foods as a contributing factor, food allergy is not a typical trigger. The rate of colic seems to be similar whether infants are breastfed or formula fed, although some studies suggest that colic is less frequent among breastfed infants. A baby with severe atopic dermatitis (eczema) and gastrointestinal symptoms like diarrhea may indeed have a food allergy and may be irritable and crying in relation to these symptoms. This is not an "otherwise healthy" infant, so this type of discomfort should not be considered true colic.

What treatments should be considered for colic?

Overall, no convincing studies prove any approach to be effective in reducing colic. Anti-gas medications do not appear to work. Reducing stimulation of the infant, according to several studies, helps 50% of infants with colic or reduces symptoms by about 50%. Some studies support dietary approaches. Any approaches to colic should be done in communication with your pediatrician or allergist.

Should the mother's diet be altered if there is colic?

Some studies show that when a breastfeeding mother avoids or reduces her consumption of milk, colic may improve whether or not there are other signs of milk allergy. Various studies have evaluated low-allergen diets, when a mother avoids typical allergenic foods (such as milk and eggs) while breastfeeding. In general, this approach was sometimes effective, but it remains unproven. Dietary changes are generally not advised as a first step in addressing colic.

Should the infant's diet be altered if there is colic?

Switching a colicky infant to a hypoallergenic infant formula may result in improved colic, whether or not there are signs of milk allergy, according to some studies. Others suggest that a lactose-free formula may be helpful. Some evidence supports using a soy formula or even an herbal tea (though feeding tea to infants can cause nutritional deficits). In general, the low-allergen diet was effective, but only about one-half to one-third as effective as reducing stimulation (see above). Dietary changes are generally unproved as treatments for colic and are not a first step.

What dietary approaches are suggested for colic if reduced stimulation doesn't work?
Although studies are lacking, some suggest treatment with reduced stimulation and then, if needed, a weeklong trial on a low-allergen diet. In any event, a link to allergy has not been proven. Colic improves spontaneously, so luckily there is an end in sight even if these dietary measures do not seem to work.

What is constipation?
Constipation has symptoms that may include infrequent bowel movements, hard stools, and painful defecation. There are a huge number of potential causes, including diet, medications, diseases of the bowel, and psychological issues.

Is constipation due to food allergy?
A few studies link milk allergy to constipation that has not responded to other measures. By far, however, most cases of constipation are not related to food allergies.

How is diet related to constipation?
Talk to your doctor if you are experiencing constipation. Dietary measures, such as increasing fiber or liquids, may be recommended.

What is reflux?
Also known as gastroesophageal reflux disease (GERD), or acid reflux, this illness occurs when stomach acid comes up into the esophagus, the tube connecting the mouth and stomach. Symptoms can include heartburn, cough, chest pain, and pain with or trouble swallowing. The acid can burn the esophagus and may come up into the throat and nose, causing asthma, hoarseness, tooth decay, sinus troubles, and chronic damage to the esophagus.

What causes reflux?

Reflux is usually attributed to problems that make it easier for food and acid to make it up past the valve that usually prevents a backwash from the stomach. For example, there may be a physical problem with this valve, or obesity may lead to increased pressure, or medications or illnesses may reduce the strength of the valve. There may be overproduction of stomach acid as well.

Is reflux due to food allergy?

Reflux is usually not caused by food allergies, although a few studies have shown a link for some people, especially to milk in children. Another illness that is a concern with reflux symptoms is eosinophilic esophagitis, an allergic disorder often associated with food allergies. This illness sometimes mimics reflux, but certain symptoms differentiate it, as described later in this chapter.

Proctocolitis (Food Protein–Induced Proctocolitis)

My infant has mucousy, bloody stools. Is this a food allergy?

It may be a food allergy called food protein–induced proctocolitis.

What is proctocolitis?

Proctocolitis, or food protein–induced allergic proctocolitis, is the name of a food allergy affecting infants that causes the stool to have mucous and blood. It is most often diagnosed in breastfed babies. These babies are otherwise well, are growing normally, do not have other symptoms, and do not become anemic because the amount of blood lost is usually small.

Is food allergy the only reason a baby might have bloody or mucousy stools?

No. This symptom can also result from infections, anatomical problems such as blockages, or minor irritations such as small tears in the anus. Babies with proctocolitis have stool with small amounts of mucous and blood mixed in, whereas some of the other problems may result in diarrhea (infection) or a small bit of blood on the surface of a stool (tear). If you see blood in the stool, talk to your doctor; do not assume it is proctocolitis.

What causes proctocolitis?

Proctocolitis is a minor allergic response to a protein, such as cow's milk protein in infant formulas or passed in the mother's breast milk. The illness is generally mild, and the baby is otherwise well. If a biopsy is performed, a small amount of allergic inflammation is seen in the rectum, but a biopsy is rarely needed.

What foods trigger proctocolitis?

By far the most common trigger is cow's milk. Other potential causes include eggs, soy, wheat, and others.

How is proctocolitis treated?

For breastfed infants, the mother is usually instructed to avoid or reduce cow's milk in her diet. The bleeding should stop within a few days. If it continues, other foods may be avoided, and the doctor may look harder for other causes.

Does the mother of an infant with proctocolitis have to strictly avoid the food?

Not necessarily. When first removing a food from the diet, it should be removed strictly to see if the bleeding responds. After that, the mother may be able to have small amounts in her diet without producing symptoms in the infant.

Does food protein–induced proctocolitis go away?

Yes.

How long does it take for food protein–induced proctocolitis to resolve?

Depending on how severe the symptoms were, tests for resolution might be made in weeks or a few months after the symptoms respond to dietary elimination. The course of resolution has not been studied adequately, but proctocolitis is usually resolved by the time an infant is 1 year old. Some studies suggest that a virus is often the true cause of bleeding, which provides evidence for reintroducing the suspected trigger food sooner to see if the bleeding is truly related to the food. Another reason to retry the food in just a few weeks or months after the bleeding has stopped is that prolonged avoidance of allergens could be associated with a higher risk of developing a food allergy (see chapter 9).

How do you know if food protein–induced proctocolitis has resolved?

Your physician will simply instruct you to gradually add milk (or other trigger foods) to your diet if you are still breastfeeding or to the infant's diet. If you see blood reappear, then avoidance is resumed until the next trial.

Do infants with proctocolitis go on to have other food allergies?

They may. A single study conducted in 2020 suggested a possible higher risk. Having proctocolitis and eczema together might be even higher risk.

Food Protein–Induced Enterocolitis Syndrome

My infant had severe vomiting two hours after a meal, became pale and sleepy, and later had diarrhea. Is that a food allergy?

It may be a food allergy called food protein–induced enterocolitis syndrome (FPIES).

What is FPIES?

This is a serious food allergy that usually starts in infancy. The symptoms are severe vomiting and diarrhea. Unlike typical food allergies, there are no hives or wheezing, and allergy tests by skin or blood are negative.

How would I know if my infant has FPIES?

There is a typical pattern of symptoms that differ depending on whether the food has been a consistent part of the diet or was ingested after a period of avoidance. FPIES is often initially misdiagnosed as an infection, with consideration of a food allergy coming up when repeated symptoms are noted from reintroduction of the trigger foods.

What are the symptoms of FPIES when a baby is routinely eating the food that causes the reaction?

The infant will have increasing vomiting and diarrhea, and may appear pale and lethargic. He or she can seem very ill, and physicians might suspect a serious infection or surgical problem.

What are the symptoms of FPIES from first ingestion of a food or from reintroducing it after not eating it for a time?

The infant or young child appears perfectly well for about 1 to 3 hours but then begins to vomit, often profusely and repetitively. The child may become pale or blue in color and lethargic, with low blood pressure. Several hours later, there is often diarrhea. The illness looks very much like a severe infection. If a blood test is performed, there may be a large number of cells called neutrophils and a high number of platelets, another blood component. The blood test results may lead a doctor to further suspect infection.

What foods cause FPIES?

The most common foods are milk and soy. When grains are responsible, usually oat or rice is the allergen. Many different foods have been found to trigger this response in children.

What are the chances that a baby with milk FPIES will react to other foods?

This varies a lot among study findings, but roughly half of these children react to soy, and about a quarter of them react to a solid food, such as oat or rice.

What are the chances that a baby with rice or oat FPIES will react to other solids?

More than half the patients with FPIES in our referral center react to more than one food, with about two-thirds reacting to milk or soy and about half reacting to another grain (not usually wheat). These percentages have been much lower in studies from other countries. It means that advancing the diet requires care and working with an allergist.

How is FPIES treated?

The only current treatment is to avoid the trigger foods.

Why does FPIES happen?

The immune system responds to trigger foods by releasing chemicals affecting the gut and circulation. These are somewhat different from those that are released in anaphylaxis. IgE is not involved.

How is an FPIES reaction treated?

The primary treatment is to avoid the trigger food. But if the food is eaten and a reaction occurs, the child should be given fluids. Because blood pressure is often low, and the child is vomiting, fluids are given through a vein (intravenously, an IV) under medical supervision. Therefore treatment in an emergency room is required. The reaction is thought to be due to immune cells, so treatment with steroids to quell immune cells is also usually given, but this treatment is not proved. A medication called ondansetron (brand name Zofran) may help relieve vomiting, although more studies are needed. This medicine is usually prescribed to treat vomiting caused by chemotherapy treatments and viral illnesses, and it has to be used cautiously in people with a certain type of uncommon heart disease called "prolonged QT." Medicines used for anaphylaxis, such as epinephrine and antihistamines, are not typically used as treatments for FPIES. Severely ill children may receive additional medications in the hospital to help regulate blood pressure.

Should a child with FPIES have epinephrine available?

An epinephrine autoinjector is not routinely recommended.

Are there different severities of FPIES?

Yes. An FPIES reaction may be mild, with just a small amount of vomiting, or severe, with all the symptoms described above.

Can FPIES be fatal?

Thus far, there have been no recorded deaths attributed to FPIES.

How do you approach feeding new foods to a baby who has FPIES?

Because there is currently no simple test to predict a reaction, introduction of the most common triggers (milk, soy, oat, rice) is often delayed until the infant is age 1 year or older. We do not know if there is any benefit to waiting longer, or possibly trying sooner, however, so this time frame should be individualized with your allergist. Some foods are only rarely associated with FPIES, and so they might be tried earlier. Table 5.2 categorizes foods by risk based upon several studies reporting trigger foods, which may also reflect typical timing of some of these foods (trials of earlier infant foods may be associated with more reactions to them). As egg and peanut are being encouraged as earlier foods for infants, we may be seeing more cases of FPIES in them.

Table 5.2. Risk Categories of Example Foods for FPIES

High	Medium	Low	Lowest
Milk	Egg	Banana	Apple
Oat	Fish	Barley	Berries
Rice	Peanut	Beef	Broccoli
Soy	Poultry	Legumes	Cauliflower
		Sweet potato	Orange
		Wheat	Pear
			Quinoa
			Turnip

How are decisions about introducing new foods made for infants with FPIES?

Introducing a new food for an infant with FPIES can be complicated. Your allergist has to decide whether foods can be tried at home or should be introduced under supervision, and when. The timing of introducing risky foods might vary depending on the severity of past reactions—waiting longer, for example, if past reactions were severe. The decisions are also based on epidemiology, or the risk for particular foods. Introducing oat or rice for the first time to an infant who already reacted to milk and soy is riskier than trying other foods (fruits, vegetables, meats, and other grains). If an infant had reactions to foods that are rare triggers (fruits, sweet potatoes, other vegetables), going slower and cautiously with more introductions under supervision would be warranted.

Does FPIES resolve?

In most cases it does.

How is an infant or child tested to see if FPIES has resolved?

By a feeding test. Allergy skin or blood tests are not helpful in identifying whether the problem resolved.

How long does it take for FPIES to go away?

It is difficult to test for resolution because a feeding test is needed. The problem appears to resolve in one to three years in most cases.

Can a baby with FPIES develop "regular" food allergies?

Yes, about 10% of the time, especially to milk. Even though typical tests for allergies do not give any information about whether FPIES has resolved, they might be performed to determine whether typical anaphylactic allergies have developed.

What should I do if my child is having symptoms or has eaten a food that triggered FPIES in the past?

You should go to the emergency room even before the symptoms start, if possible. Since many doctors are not familiar with FPIES, I suggest carrying a letter that explains the illness. Here is an example letter:

> Dear Doctor [or To Whom It May Concern],
>
> My child has a food allergy called food protein–induced enterocolitis syndrome. This is a type of allergy that usually does not result in typical allergic symptoms such as hives or wheezing; instead, it has isolated gastrointestinal symptoms.
>
> The foods that my child is avoiding include:_____. The symptoms of this type of allergic reaction include repetitive vomiting, which may not start until a few (e.g., 2) hours following ingestion of the food to which my child is allergic. Even trace amounts can trigger a reaction. There is often diarrhea that starts later (after 6 hours). In some cases (~20%), the reaction includes hypotension and lethargy, sometimes acidemia and methemoglobinemia. The treatment is symptomatic and can include intravenous fluids (e.g., normal saline bolus, hydration) and steroids for significant symptoms. The latter is given because the pathophysiology is that of a T-cell response. Ondansetron (Zofran) may also be helpful, particularly intravenously.
>
> This information is being given for consideration in the differential diagnosis of my child in the event of symptoms. Of course, my child having this illness does not preclude the possibility of other illnesses (e.g., infection, toxic ingestion, etc.) or even other types of allergic reactions leading to symptoms, so it is up to the evaluating physician to consider all possibilities. Similarly, the treating physician

is encouraged to pursue any other treatments deemed necessary (e.g., symptomatic, such as epinephrine for shock, antibiotics for presumed infection, etc.).

Sincerely,
Your name [or your doctor's name]

The letter has a lot of "doctor speak," which I will decode: *acidemia* is increased acid in the blood, *hypotension* is low blood pressure, *T-cells* are mentioned to explain that this is not an IgE antibody–related allergy, and *methemoglobinemia* is a response that results in blue color of the skin.

Can a breastfed baby have FPIES from food eaten by the mother?
This happens rarely. If it does, the mother must avoid eating the causal food.

Does a mother who is breastfeeding need to avoid the food that triggered FPIES in her infant when the baby ate the food directly?
We do not have studies that compare outcomes whether a mother avoids the food or not. Assuming the infant is otherwise doing well, I do not usually have a mother avoid the culprit food, but I may advise her not to exceed the amounts she has usually eaten while the infant has been well.

How much food must be eaten by an infant or child to trigger an FPIES reaction?
Similar to typical allergies, some children may be sensitive to trace amounts, and others might not react until ingesting a larger amount. There is no test to determine how sensitive a child might be. Sometimes we see a child tolerate an increasing amount prior to having symptoms as they outgrow the allergy.

Can an FPIES reaction be triggered from touch or smell?
No.

Can FPIES occur in adults?
Yes, but it is uncommon. It may occur because an allergy was never outgrown (rare). When FPIES occurs in adults, the most common trigger is seafood.

Does FPIES run in families?

There are insufficient studies to know for certain, but siblings may have a higher risk of having FPIES.

Food Protein Enteropathy and Protein Intolerance

What is food protein enteropathy?

This is an uncommon illness of infants, with some symptoms similar to celiac disease (diarrhea, poor growth, and low protein, or loss of protein in the gut). There can be swelling of the face and body because of protein imbalances. If a gastroenterologist does a biopsy, inflammation is seen in the gut. Unlike celiac, this illness resolves. The common triggers are milk or soy.

What is food protein intolerance?

The term "food protein intolerance" is not defined in any specific way; it is not a medical diagnosis. It is sometimes used to describe FPIES, eosinophilic gastroenteropathy, or nonspecific gastrointestinal symptoms that are attributed to foods.

Eosinophilic Esophagitis and Other Eosinophilic Gut Diseases

What is an eosinophil?

An eosinophil is a cell of the immune system that is prominent in the allergic inflammation that causes asthma and chronic allergic inflammation in the gut.

Sometimes food gets stuck in my throat or hurts going down after being swallowed. Can this be a food allergy?

This symptom is a common one in older children and adults who have eosinophilic esophagitis, an illness often related to food allergies.

What is eosinophilic esophagitis?

This is a chronic illness in which allergic inflammation, comprising eosinophils, occurs in the esophagus, the tube that squeezes food from the mouth into the stomach. The esophagus is the most common location of this type of inflammation in the gut. The illness is tough to treat because it is like having a rash inside the body. It is hard to know what is triggering inflammation or how it responds to treatments. Some people may develop scarring that seriously affects their ability to eat.

What is eosinophilic gastritis?

This illness is usually associated with eosinophilic esophagitis, and it also involves chronic allergic inflammation, but in the stomach. The main symptoms are nausea and stomach pain.

What is eosinophilic gastroenteritis?

In this illness, allergic inflammation occurs all along the gut, and symptoms include pain, poor growth, vomiting, and diarrhea. There can be swelling of the face and body due to protein loss in the gut, leading to protein imbalances. Treatment often requires elimination of multiple foods. As with eosinophilic esophagitis (described below), it is difficult to identify exactly which foods are problematic in people with eosinophilic gastroenteritis. The natural course of the illness is not well studied.

What are typical symptoms of eosinophilic esophagitis?

Common symptoms include abdominal pain, nausea/vomiting, heartburn, and swallowing difficulty. The inflammation swells the esophagus, making it hard for it to do its job of squeezing food down to the stomach. Therefore there is pain with food going down, or the food may not go down at all and get stuck. People with this illness may chew their food for a long time and drink a lot of water with meals to compensate for the problem. When there is vomiting, it may be mucousy and sticky because of the chemicals released from the allergy cells. There can be heartburn symptoms as well. If food gets stuck going down, there may be drooling because the esophagus is blocked. This feeling might mimic anaphylaxis. Young children may have poor growth.

What causes eosinophilic esophagitis?

There appears to be an inherited disposition to having inflammation in the esophagus. The usual triggers seem to be allergens.

How common is eosinophilic esophagitis?
This illness appears to affect as many as 1 in 1,000.

Does eosinophilic esophagitis run in families?
Yes.

Who is at risk for eosinophilic esophagitis?
People with food and other allergies or with a history of eosinophilic esophagitis in the family are at risk. The illness is more common in boys.

At what age is eosinophilic esophagitis usually diagnosed?
The typical ages of diagnosis are during childhood or among adults in their 30s and 40s. The illness can occur in all age groups, however, including infants.

How is eosinophilic esophagitis diagnosed?
Symptoms of vomiting, pain, reflux (heartburn), and especially food getting stuck while swallowing may raise suspicion. A biopsy, performed by putting a tube down the esophagus, is used to diagnose this disease and whether it is responding to therapies.

Are biopsies dangerous?
No. After the person is asleep from the medications, a tube with a camera (endoscope) is put down the esophagus. The esophagus is inspected for signs of inflammation (like a rash), and small "bites" of the surface are taken for checking under a microscope. The procedure is generally over in about 20 minutes, and the risks are minimal (including anesthesia risks and the risk of bleeding or tearing the esophagus, which are extremely uncommon).

What role does food allergy play in eosinophilic esophagitis?
In studies of children, food is usually shown to be a trigger. For some people, allergens in the air, such as pollens, are important causes, and for others, the inflammation has no obvious trigger. In adults, the relationship between foods and eosinophilic esophagitis has not been tested as thoroughly, but foods probably play a role.

Can removal of food allergens improve eosinophilic esophagitis?
Yes, but often many foods are triggers.

How do you determine which foods are triggering eosinophilic esophagitis?

Suspicions about food triggers are addressed based on personal history, knowledge about common food triggers, testing, elimination diets, food challenges, and biopsies. The primary way to determine whether a particular food is a trigger is to remove it from the diet and then perform a biopsy to see if the inflammation improved. Or, if inflammation was under control after some dietary changes were made, another biopsy could be performed after a food was introduced to see if it was tolerated or if it triggered inflammation. This is a tedious process because multiple foods might be triggers.

What are the common food triggers for eosinophilic esophagitis?

The major allergens that cause sudden allergic reactions are triggers, especially milk and wheat but also eggs, fish, peanuts, shellfish, soy, and tree nuts. Triggers for eosinophilic esophagitis also include beef, corn, and many others.

What role do allergy tests play in diagnosing food allergies in eosinophilic esophagitis?

Only a minimal one. Although allergy tests are often performed, they do not correlate well with identifying the true triggers, so trials of dietary avoidance are usually needed. Allergy blood tests, skin prick tests, and even patch tests (see chapter 3) might be used, but none have proven reliability for this illness. They may be used as guides.

How important are elimination diets and feeding tests in diagnosing eosinophilic esophagitis?

Eliminating targeted foods to watch for resolution of symptoms and improvement in biopsies as well as performing food challenges followed by biopsies and observation are the main approaches to diagnosing food triggers in eosinophilic esophagitis. There are many possible approaches, such as removing one or many foods and waiting for a response over subsequent weeks; making a diet that includes only a list of foods that are probably safe based on the person's history and test results; or using a diet that relies on the nonallergenic amino acid–based formula. The approaches to trial diets are summarized in table 5.3.

Table 5.3. Common Types of Trial Elimination Diets for Eosinophilic Esophagitis

Type of Diet	Details	Risk/Benefit
Elemental diet	Use only a nonallergenic formula	Will work (effectiveness of more than 90%) if the illness is caused by any food, but the diet is too difficult for long-term practicality
Diet based on testing	Remove foods that are tested positive	The tests do not reflect triggers well. Should remove milk even if test is negative. If only a few foods test positive, this diet might be less burdensome. Works about 50% to 70% of the time.
Four-food elimination diet	Egg, milk, soy, wheat	May have good effect with few foods. Works about 50% to 70% of the time.
Six-food elimination diet (really more than six)	Adds peanut/tree nut, fish/shellfish (some include legumes)	As above
Milk and/or wheat	Initial diet might remove milk only, wheat only, or both	Removing the most common trigger (milk) or the top two might be most likely to have improvement with the least amount of initial elimination

How are medications used to treat eosinophilic esophagitis?

The most effective therapy currently is steroids. Giving regular doses of steroids—for example, by giving pills or injections—carries side effects. Current treatment is aimed at trying to coat the esophagus with steroids, similar to putting a cream on a rash. The person swallows a form of steroids that is usually found in asthma inhalers. Studies are ongoing for promising new therapies, such as injected or oral treatments that reduce eosinophils.

Should diet changes or medications be used to treat eosinophilic esophagitis?

This is often based on personal preference and trial and error, seeing what works better and what is less stressful to do. Often, a combination approach is used.

What are the risks of diet treatment of eosinophilic esophagitis?

The diet may be limited, carrying social and nutritional consequences. Rarely, a food removed from the diet may trigger a sudden allergic reaction when reintroduced. A dietitian may be needed to provide nutritional advice if many foods are eliminated.

What are the risks of medical treatment of eosinophilic esophagitis?

The steroids can cause localized dryness and an increased risk of fungal infection in the esophagus or mouth and throat. This risk can be reduced by rinsing the mouth and brushing after taking the treatment. In small doses, the medication should not affect growth, but growth monitoring is recommended for children. Doctors aim to use the least amount needed to get results.

Why does eosinophilic esophagitis need to be treated?

Two reasons. First, the illness is uncomfortable, and treatment should address the symptoms. Second, if the inflammation is left unchecked, there could be scarring.

How serious is the risk of scarring in eosinophilic esophagitis?

Some persons with this illness develop scarring that constricts the esophagus, and they require a procedure that stretches the tube to let food down, a procedure that may need to be performed periodically. Biopsies may detect scarring early, but we do not yet know who gets scarring, how quickly it happens, and whether treating it early totally reverses it. This situation, when treatment improves symptoms but leaves some degree of inflammation, is frustrating. It is not totally clear whether the inflammation and scarring may also increase the risk of cancer of the esophagus.

How does one know when eosinophilic esophagitis is being treated properly?

When symptoms are improved and a biopsy shows that the inflammation is resolved or substantially lessened.

Will eosinophilic esophagitis go away?

This illness appears to be persistent and chronic for most people affected.

Besides diet and steroids, are there other treatments on the horizon?

Active research is being done on treatments that might better reduce the inflammation, such as injected antibodies that disable eosinophils, the main problem in this illness. Other antiallergy treatments, such as antihistamines, and medications called cromolyn and antileukotrienes have been evaluated without significant success. There is also research into ways to better diagnose eosinophilic esophagitis without having to do biopsies.

Is eosinophilic esophagitis treatable with anti-reflux medications?

A trial of stomach acid–blocking medications is often recommended because sometimes this treatment is all that is needed to reverse the inflammation.

Chronic Illnesses That Are Not Related to Food Allergies

Why do some people say that chronic problems like arthritis, autism, epilepsy, headaches, and hyperactivity are caused by food allergies?

There are theories that foods play a role in many illnesses, and people often use the term "allergy" when talking about this connection. The word "allergy" actually refers to immune responses, so most of the theories should not be using the term "food allergy." Some theories hold that chemicals in milk or wheat play a role in autism, but I am not aware of any studies that confirm this relationship, and scientists have mostly concluded there is no clear relationship. Studies are ongoing to evaluate the role of diet in autism. Nonetheless, there does not appear to be an allergy involved, not even in the theories as described.

Epilepsy (seizure) treatment has been approached with removal of allergens from the diet without clear effect or clear reasoning to support the approach. Some types of seizure disorders, however, respond to a special type of "starvation" diet, which has nothing to do with allergies. Regarding headaches, it is thought that some dietary components, especially tyramine or similar chemicals and perhaps natural histamines—found in foods such as banana, bouillon, canned meat, cheese, chocolate, pickled herring, soy sauce, and wine—are able to trigger migraines in some sensitive persons. Some literature links rheumatoid arthritis flares to foods. The relationship is unproven, but if it does exist, it may have to do with the inflammatory aspects of the foods, such as a lack of healthful fatty acids. Regarding behavioral problems, childhood hyperactivity has been related to chemical food additives in some children. These issues are discussed in chapter 1 as well.

Delving Deeper

Should allergy skin testing or blood testing be done for FPIES?

When children or adults have classical symptoms of delayed repetitive vomiting and other symptoms of FPIES and no symptoms of typical anaphylactic allergies, like having hives, the allergy tests for IgE to the trigger food are almost always negative. Allergists may want to perform the tests for several reasons. The allergist may want to "prove" there is no evidence of IgE. This could allay concerns that there is an unusual gut-only reaction that upon re-exposure might instead result in typical allergic reactions. Another reason may be to follow up on the allergy after a period of avoidance. Some children may begin to show positive tests and then have typical allergic reactions. This has primarily been an issue with milk. The delay in onset of symptoms with FPIES characteristically occurs within two to three hours. This is slower than typical IgE-mediated allergy but faster than symptoms from alpha-gal allergy. There may be some people with alpha-gal allergy (from tick bites) who primarily have gut symptoms that may mimic FPIES (although usually milder), and in this case an IgE test may be helpful.

How common is it for a new allergy to develop if we eliminate foods for treating eosinophilic esophagitis or atopic dermatitis?

There is no clear answer because there are few studies about this topic. For eosinophilic esophagitis, milk seems to be a particular issue. Just a few reports describe children or adults who avoided milk and then became allergic or at least developed positive tests (see Hill et al. and Ho and Chehade in chapter 11). The individuals were typically allergy-prone, with eczema, and were avoiding milk for more than a year. One child who had resolved a milk allergy at age 3 years redeveloped it at age 14 years, with re-exposure after 4 months off milk to treat the eosinophilic esophagitis (see Soller et al. in chapter 11). Overall, this is an uncommon issue in eosinophilic esophagitis but should be considered and monitored.

For atopic dermatitis, there were reports from the early 1980s describing anaphylaxis in children who were put on elimination diets to treat their eczema, when they again tried previously avoided foods. A study from 2016 (see Chang et al. in chapter 11) evaluated 132 children where food allergy was considered a trigger of the rash. More than two years later, 40% had experienced immediate-type allergic reactions, with about half never having had that happen before. About one in five allergic reactions was to foods the child had been eating previously. In summary, a significant number of children could have allergies to foods eliminated to treat their eczema, and so a careful discussion about risks and benefits of dietary approaches and medical approaches is important in making decisions about care.

CHAPTER 6

Mastering Allergen Avoidance

In this chapter, I answer questions about avoiding allergic reactions and managing food allergies at home, when shopping, when dining out, in school, at camps, at work, when traveling, and in other settings.

General Questions about Avoiding Allergic Reactions

What do I need to know to keep myself and others safe from food allergens?

It is necessary to think about allergen avoidance at every meal and social circumstance. Knowledge about cross-contact and reading labels are key. You may feel overwhelmed by everything you need to know, but reading this chapter should help. Accidents can happen, but being prepared and educated can go a long way in maintaining safety.

What are some common mistakes people make when avoiding a food allergen?

Accidental exposures to avoided allergens often occur when people drop their guard, not thinking about or assuming the safety of a food. Constant vigilance is needed to consider the safety of foods at each meal and snack. Ingredient labels must be read carefully. When others offer a food, they must understand about food allergies and how to create a "safe" meal. Mistakes also occur from failure to recognize cross-contact of allergens into otherwise safe foods.

How do I avoid the common mistakes in avoiding food allergens?

Educate yourself and others, and always stay vigilant!

If I am curious whether my or my child's allergy has resolved, is it all right to try a small amount of the food?

NO! Always talk to your allergist if you are curious or suspect an allergy has waned or resolved. Testing and possibly a doctor-supervised feeding test may be warranted, but do not try this at home.

Is it a good strategy to assess the safety of a food with a small bite, checking for mouth itch?

This is a potentially dangerous approach that is sometimes wrongly used to bypass asking meaningful questions about ingredients and food preparation. The strategy is faulty because often there is no mouth itch prior to having a severe reaction. A taste test is also unreliable because if there is an allergen in part of a food or meal, the initial bite might not contain it. Additionally, the small taste may not evoke a symptom, but a larger amount, when eaten, could. If any antihistamines are being used to treat allergies, these would also reduce or eliminate any mouth symptoms. For all of these reasons, never use this approach to assess the safety of a meal or food.

Is it possible to use a laboratory or test kit to check if a food has an allergen?

Some commercial laboratory tests and some "quick tests" (designed like a urine pregnancy test, scanners, and other devices) detect specific food proteins, such as those in peanuts. Commercial manufacturers might use these tests to check if they have sufficiently cleaned their equipment between running an allergen-containing and an allergen-free product. An increasing number of consumer products to quickly detect allergens in meals are entering the market. So far, we have not seen fully dependable devices. Typically, a small bit of the food is tested, and the allergen could be in some other part of the food. It remains vital to ask good questions, follow recommended ways to obtain safe foods, and check product ingredient labels carefully, as described below.

Cross-Contact

What is cross-contact?

Cross-contact, sometimes called cross-contamination, happens when an otherwise allergen-safe food contains an unintentional allergen because of an error during cooking or preparing the food.

What are common examples of allergen cross-contact?

- A knife used to spread peanut butter is placed into the jelly jar. Now the jelly jar has some peanut in it that may be introduced into an otherwise-safe jelly sandwich at another time.
- A spatula used to loosen some nut-containing cookies from a pan is then used to serve nut-free cookies, introducing nuts onto those cookies.
- French fries are made in a fryer that cooked fried shrimp and fish sticks. Now the French fries have fish and shellfish proteins on them.
- A hamburger is fried on a skillet where a cheeseburger was cooked, introducing milk onto the hamburger.
- A shake mixer is used to make a peanut-flavored milkshake. A peanut-free milkshake is now blended with the same mixer that was not cleaned, introducing peanut into the peanut-free milkshake.
- A wok used for cashew chicken is now used to heat beef and broccoli, introducing nut proteins into that dish.
- Nuts are chopped on a cutting board that is next used to chop lettuce for a nut-free salad, introducing nut proteins into the salad.
- A mixing spoon used to stir cream soup is next used to stir vegetable soup, introducing milk into the milk-free soup.
- A food handler does not change gloves as she touches a food allergen and then handles food that was intended to be allergen-free.

How does one avoid cross-contact?

There has to be an ongoing consciousness about cross-contact to maintain a safe supply of allergen-free ingredients for meals. This may be possible in a home where family members know that they need to take care to keep ingredients allergen-free at all times. It may be unlikely to occur in places where there is not a constant need to maintain an allergen-free source of ingredients, such as in restaurants, bakeries, or homes without allergic individuals. Therefore, depending on the circumstances, there may be a need for ongoing vigilance (at home) or for education on how to make individual meals that are allergen-safe (for restaurants, friends' homes, and so on).

In an ice cream shop, is washing the scoop sufficient to avoid an allergen?

No. If the scoop was previously used in several ice cream containers, there could already be cross-contact of allergens in the ice cream tubs. For example, if the patron before you ordered a double scoop of vanilla and peanut, the peanut might already have been spread into the vanilla. A clean scoop used in the vanilla would not alter the contamination. An alternative is to ask for a clean scoop and to open a new tub of the ice cream.

What are some tips to avoid cross-contact with allergens?

Keep foods covered in cupboards and refrigerators. Make the safe food for the person with allergies and set it aside before making foods that contain the allergen. Teach others to avoid the pitfalls described above.

Amounts That Trigger a Reaction and Casual Exposure

How much food needs to be eaten to trigger a reaction?

The amount of food that can trigger a reaction depends on an individual's sensitivity. It is not easily predicted by any simple tests. For some people, trace amounts that are not easily visible to the naked eye may cause symptoms, while for others, a meal-size amount of a food or more may be required to trigger a reaction. Your doctor may be able to assess your level of sensitivity based on your history or your response to a feeding test. Studies have tried to determine the lowest amount that would trigger symptoms (not necessarily severe ones) in the top 10% of sensitive people. For foods like egg, milk, peanut, sesame, and tree nuts, the amounts are in the range of about 3–10 milligrams (see Ballmer-Weber et al. in chapter 11). Different foods and preparations of them have differing protein content, but this would look something like a half a drop of milk, one-hundredth of a peanut kernel or of a cashew kernel, and about five sesame seeds.

Can smelling a food cause an allergic reaction?

Yes, but this type of exposure is unlikely to cause anaphylaxis.

When can smelling a food cause an allergic reaction?

When the protein from the food is distributed into the air.

Under what circumstances would food proteins become airborne?

This most often occurs from heating, such as in cooking. For example, the steam from scrambling eggs or frying fish and the vapor from boiling or frothing milk can carry proteins into the air. Another way proteins can get into the air is when the food is in a powdery form and gets disturbed, for example, when preparing foods with wheat flour, powdered milk, or dried egg powder. Last, manipulations of a food might spread some proteins into the air nearby, for example, when peeling an orange or cracking peanuts.

In what settings might there be an abundance of food proteins in the air?

Examples include occupational settings, such as a bakery or food-processing factory; markets where a high concentration of the food is being processed or heated, such as a seafood market; food stands or kitchen locations where foods are being heated, such as roasting nuts or frothing milk at a coffee shop.

Is smelling a food likely to cause an allergic reaction?

Rarely. Most smells from foods are due to organic compounds and contain no appreciable proteins. For example, the smell of peanut butter is not from any significant protein in the air. Odors from foods that are not being actively heated are unlikely to expel any appreciable allergenic proteins.

What kinds of symptoms might happen from airborne food proteins?

The symptoms would be similar to those from allergens such as pollens and animal danders. Namely, there may be itchy eyes, sneezing, a runny nose, and, for people with asthma, a cough or wheeze.

Can touching a food cause an allergic reaction?

Yes, but anaphylaxis is unlikely.

What kinds of symptoms might happen from touching a food?

The most common skin symptoms are red blotches, hives, and itchiness. But touching the food does not usually cause symptoms. The skin barrier prevents the proteins from reaching the immune system. Younger children are often more susceptible to skin reactions from direct contact, especially if their skin barrier is compromised by eczema rashes. The eyes are also sensitive to allergens, so an allergen from the fingers rubbed into the eyes can result in significant redness and swelling. Contact to food allergens on skin that is rashy, for example, from eczema, could result in stronger reactions because the skin barrier is disrupted.

Can a severe reaction happen from touching or smelling a food?

Rarely. If a person with asthma breathes in a large inhalation of a food allergen, a significant asthma attack might occur. If a large area of abraded skin is exposed to an allergen, there may be more absorption, leading to stronger reactions. However, these are unusual circumstances. The primary concern about casual exposure to a food is transferring the food from fingers into the mouth.

How worried should I be that my child will touch or smell an allergen and develop an allergic reaction?

Anxiety and controversy surround the worry that smelling or touching an allergen could result in a severe allergic reaction. Although there are examples of foods becoming airborne during cooking or when they are in a powdery form, the risks should be taken in context. A study that purposefully aerosolized foods to which a child was allergic by cooking them found no reactions or primarily mild ones (see Roberts and Lack in chapter 11). Our studies in which peanut-allergic children smelled or were touched by peanut butter resulted in no reactions or in mild redness at the site of contact (see Simonte et al. in chapter 11). There is reason to have concern, but the anxiety about these exposures is probably greater than the actual risks warrant. Talk to your doctor about the risks. Your allergist might suggest a "test" of touching or smelling a food to address your concerns.

What are some surprising mistakes that have led to allergic reactions?

Our studies showed that sometimes parents or other family members fed an allergen purposefully to a child with allergies, or allergic individuals purposefully ate foods they were allergic to, resulting in reactions (Fleischer et al. 2012; see chapter 11). The reasons for this include curiosity, thinking a small amount would be okay, and testing to see if the allergy had resolved. If you are unsure you have an allergy, always discuss this with your doctor before trying an allergen at home. Teach caretakers the same.

Is it okay for a person with egg allergy to color Easter eggs?
Yes, but carefully. The most potent part of egg is the white, and raw egg is the most potent form of egg allergen. Sometimes the surface of the egg has the egg white on it, and if the egg breaks, there will be an even larger exposure. The skin contact isn't likely to trigger a significant reaction, but doing a craft project with the eggs and then rubbing egg-white-laden fingers into the eye could induce swelling. Participation might include using plastic eggs, wearing gloves, or being careful not to place your fingers in your eyes or mouth.

Can a person with tree nut allergy be near oak trees with acorns?
Acorns are tree nuts, and they might be allergens if eaten, but they are too sour to eat, so there is no literature about reactions from eating them. Like other nuts, it is not likely that touching them would result in any significant allergic reactions.

Can a person with seafood allergy swim in the ocean?
Yes. I am not aware of any reports of a person being allergic to seawater based on an allergy to fish or shellfish. This is probably true for several reasons. First, the dilution of proteins in the ocean is so tremendous that the concentration of allergenic protein in the water becomes irrelevant. Second, the allergenic proteins in fish or shellfish are muscle proteins that would not be directly leaching into the water.

Can a person with a fish allergy own pet fish?
Yes, since the allergenic proteins are inside the fish and are not being eaten. However, the fish food is often made of fish and shellfish. If you are handling the food, minimize skin exposure by tapping the food into the water from a cap or container and washing your hands afterward. The main risk here might be rubbing the fish food on your hand into the eye, causing swelling.

Can a person with a fish allergy go fishing?
Yes, although handling the fish or handling parts of the fish after cleaning could irritate the skin because of localized allergic reactions. The main risk would be of skin or eye reactions, and possibly ingestion reactions if there is transfer to the mouth. It is possible to enjoy fishing by reducing direct handling of the fish, rinsing hands afterward, and wearing gloves when possible.

Can a person with a seafood allergy go to a dolphin show or swim with dolphins?

Dolphins themselves do not have allergenic fish proteins because they are mammals, but they eat fish and swim in an enclosed area where the dilution is less than that in the ocean. Therefore there is some risk that the fish proteins they ingest are in the pool water and may cause symptoms for a person with a fish allergy, for example, if splashed.

Can a person with a food allergy swim in a pool with others who may have eaten a food that contains allergens?

When young children are snacking and swimming, there is some risk that they may share food, so supervision is needed. A better choice is not to eat while swimming. There is a risk of choking as well! The small amount of residual allergens that might be in a mouth or on the body of a person who is swimming is unlikely to be relevant to the allergic swimmer because of the dilution effect of the pool. This risk might increase if people are constantly eating in the pool and spilling food, and also if the pool is small. In most situations, however, there should be no significant concern about reacting to residual food proteins in a swimming pool.

Can a person be allergic to seawater, pool water, or any water?

Yes, but usually such allergic reactions are caused by the temperature of the water. There is a problem called cold urticaria, where swimming in cold water, or coming out of a pool and getting chilled, causes hives. It is believed to be a kind of physically induced reaction where the allergy cells respond to the change in temperature. Anaphylaxis is possible, especially with submersion in very cold water. Antihistamines are often used for treatment. Another rare illness, aquagenic urticaria, is where water of any temperature on the skin causes hives, but the person can still drink water.

Can tiny shrimp, or copepods, in drinking water cause an allergic reaction?

Get ready to become a little grossed out. There is a microscopic animal related to shrimp that lives in freshwater and sometimes in safe drinking water, especially from sources in geographic areas that have excellent natural water available for drinking. When sources of natural drinking water exceed government potability standards, the water is unfiltered, leaving these microscopic animals behind. No harmful effects have been related to these creatures.

If a cow, pig, or chicken is fed allergens such as peanut or soy, can I be allergic to that animal's meat?

This should not be a concern because the animal's meat proteins do not change based on its diet. It does not have these food proteins within its meat.

Can a person with a food allergy go shopping in a supermarket?

Although every allergen is in the store, it is not likely that allergic reactions would be elicited merely from shopping. Still, there are a few things to consider. Before seating an allergic toddler in a shopping cart, it is prudent to wipe the surfaces because it is likely that the child might suck on the handlebar or other surfaces. If there is a shellfish allergy, it may be prudent to avoid the area where seafood is being steamed, as steaming might transiently force the seafood proteins into the air.

Avoidance at Home

Does a food allergen need to be removed entirely from the home?

Usually not, but personal preferences and the ages and diets of the household members may dictate your decision. For example, if there is a person with peanut allergy in the household, and no other family member insists on eating this food, it may be easier to exclude peanut from the home since it is not a common ingredient in most foods. Conversely, most households do not restrict foods such as milk or egg because they are common components in the diet. If there are many young children with food allergies in a home, it may be easier to exclude certain ingredients to reduce the risk of unintentional sharing among the siblings. Overall, there are many options so long as care is taken for food storage, preparation, and supervision during meals.

What do people do to stay safe when they allow a food allergen in the home?

Precautions must be in place to reduce cross-contact. Keep unsafe foods away from young children who cannot self-monitor, and stay organized about knowing which foods are safe.

What are some tips for maintaining a safe home that allows the food allergen?

Consider the following checklist for safe food handling at home.

**HOME CHECKLIST TO AVOID CROSS-CONTACT
AND ACCIDENTAL EXPOSURE TO ALLERGENS**

☐ Teach all family members about cross-contact and not sharing food

☐ Prepare the allergen-safe meal ahead of those containing the allergen

☐ Specify certain shelves in cupboards or refrigerators for allergen-safe foods

☐ Specify countertop areas as "allergen-safe" for preparation of foods

☐ Use color-coding labels on purchased products and storage containers, such as green for safe and red for allergens

☐ Supervise young, food-allergic children during mealtimes to prevent sharing

☐ Keep allergenic foods out of reach of young, food-allergic children

☐ Clean dishware and utensils appropriately

☐ Do not leave foods out when young children are unsupervised

---

Does the heat of a skillet, griddle, or fryer destroy allergens?

No.

What type of cleaning is needed to remove food allergens from dishes and utensils?

Normal cleaning with soap and water should be sufficient.

Does a standard dishwasher adequately remove allergens from dishes and utensils?

Dishwashers are reliable. If the dishware and utensils appear clean after washing, without evident residue, the cleaning process is almost certain to have removed allergens.

Is it safe to cook allergen-safe foods in ovens and microwaves where allergens were cooked?

If the allergens were heated at another time, and the safe food is in a dish so that it is not in contact with the oven surfaces, there should be no problem. If the allergen is being heated in an open container along with another open container that has safe foods at the same time, there is a risk that the allergen may splatter, or that steam from the allergen may land in the safe food. Heating the foods separately or covered should allay such problems.

Is it safe to cook allergen-safe foods on grills where allergens were cooked?

If the grill is not specifically cleaned, there could be residual allergens. The heat of the grill may not destroy them. One option is to heat the allergen-safe food on aluminum foil on the grill.

Manufactured Products

What can I learn from reading a product label?

Except under unusual circumstances, the label should list all ingredients. This usually allows identification of any allergens. Surprisingly, however, some products have hidden ingredients that are not fully disclosed.

Do I need to read labels every time?

Yes. Ingredients can change, so reading the label each time ensures that you are aware of any new ingredients that could be problematic.

Is it helpful to develop a list of "safe products"?

No, it can be a dangerous practice. Ingredients change, so the list can become outdated right away. It is better practice to read the label each time.

Can ingredients vary in the same product from time to time?

Yes. Sometimes different sizes of the same product have slightly different ingredients. Sometimes a product made in one location differs somewhat from the same product manufactured in another factory. By reading the label each time, you can avoid unpleasant surprises from unexpected ingredients.

What do US food allergen–labeling laws require?

The Food Allergen Labeling and Consumer Protection Act of 2004 (FALCPA) requires that major allergens—crustacean shellfish, eggs, fish, milk, peanuts, soy, tree nuts, and wheat—that are intended ingredients in a food be listed in plain English somewhere on the ingredient label. The law applies to all packaged foods regulated under the Federal Food, Drug, and Cosmetic Act (FD&C Act). Also, the type of nut (such as almond, walnut) and species of fish (such as bass, tuna) or crustacean shellfish (such as lobster, shrimp) must be named specifically. There are various options for declaring the allergen; for example, the ingredient list might say "milk," or it might show the allergen in parentheses—"whey (milk)"—or there might be a separate line that says "Contains milk." Highly processed, refined oils that are essentially free from proteins are exempt from labeling laws. A new law was passed in 2021 to add sesame to the list starting January 2023.

Do US labeling laws apply to imported foods?

Yes, they apply to domestic and imported foods. There is a system in place to check the labeling as the shipment enters the country, and the labels can be revised, if needed. This system does not actually "test" products to verify ingredients. It just ensures that the labeling practices are following US laws.

What do the US Food and Drug Administration as well as labeling laws consider to be nuts?

Many: almond, beechnut, Brazil, butternut, cashew, chestnut, chinquapin, coconut, filbert/hazelnut, ginkgo, hickory nut, lychee nut, macadamia nut (bush nut), pecan, pili nut, pine nut/piñon, pistachio, shea nut, walnut (heartnut). Many of these are not true nuts (coconut, lychee) or pose little or no risk (shea nut butter), and revisions are being sought.

What is not covered by US labeling laws?

Any food that is not considered a major allergen, including seeds, spices, and non-crustacean seafood, such as clams and squid. Also, the laws do not currently mandate the labeling that warns of possible contamination with allergens (advisory or precautionary labeling). Egg, meat, and poultry products and other "raw" agricultural foods (fruits, vegetables, and so on) are not covered. Cosmetics and medications are not part of the laws, although allergens are often declared. Alcoholic beverages may contain allergens, including unexpected ones such as cow's milk, eggs, or seafood (used as clarifying agents). FALCPA does not cover alcoholic beverages, although the federal agency that oversees labeling of alcohol has stated an intention to apply similar rules in the near future. The relevance of allergens used as clarifying agents in wine is mostly unknown, but a couple of studies indicate no significant risk. Some countries have labeling laws that cover more foods than the US law does.

What is a "free from" statement?

Some manufacturers voluntarily label a product "free from" an allergen. They presumably do this to indicate that there is no risk of contamination, and they may be marketing their product to persons with a food allergy. There are no laws regulating this type of labeling, however.

What is a "contains" statement?

This is a separate statement, usually near the ingredients list, that discloses the major allergens in the food. This type of labeling is an option.

Can a "contains" statement show only the names of major food allergen sources that are not already identified in the ingredients list?

No. If a "contains" statement is used on a food label, it is supposed to include the names of the food sources of all major food allergens used as ingredients in the food. For example, if "egg yolks," "natural peanut flavor," and "whey" are declared in a product's ingredients list, the "contains" statement is required to identify all three sources of the major food allergens present ("Contains eggs, milk, peanuts"), not just some of them.

Will the ingredients label identify every single ingredient?

No. The label may hide some proprietary ingredients under collective labels, such as "natural flavors" or "spices." This is not the case for the major allergens included in the labeling laws.

Is there any way to find out what ingredients are in a food with ambiguous labeling such as "spices"?

It depends on the willingness of the manufacturer. I suggest that if you are interested in buying the product, you may want to pose your question in a way that does not require a full disclosure of the "secret" ingredient.

For example, you might say, "I am allergic to sesame. Is there any sesame in the spices or flavorings in your product?" If you had an allergic reaction to a food and aren't sure what caused the reaction, you should work with your doctor to get more information from the manufacturer, because it is important to track down the allergen to prevent future reactions.

What are advisory or precautionary statements?

These are voluntary statements that indicate a possible risk that an allergen could be unintentionally included in the food. There are no laws requiring these statements or guidelines on how to describe the concern, but the statements must be truthful. Manufacturers state this possibility in many different ways: "may contain _____," "made in a facility that processes _____," "made on equipment with _____," "processed in a facility that also processes _____," and many others. At this time, government agencies are considering simplifying the language used to indicate a potential risk.

Do the words used in advisory statements differentiate the degree of risk?

No. You might assume that "May contain peanuts" is riskier than "Made in a facility that also processes peanuts," but this is not the case.

How often does the product with an advisory label have the allergen in it?

Studies have shown the risk to be in the range of about 2% to 10%, but this varies by allergen and types of food (see Allen et al. in chapter 11). For example, there was a high rate of milk found in chocolate products that did not have intentional milk ingredients. Additionally, there is variation from time to time and batch to batch.

How much of the allergen might be in a product with an advisory label?

As an unintended ingredient, the amounts are typically low, but there may be enough to trigger reactions in sensitive people. Most allergists will advise avoidance of these products, but you should discuss this with your allergist in case you are not very sensitive and don't need to be as concerned.

If a product does not have an advisory label, does that mean there is no risk?
Technically, no. Since advisory labeling is voluntary, an unintended ingredient could be in a food without a warning.

How often would a product without an advisory warning contain an allergen?
Studies (see Ford et al. and Hefle et al. in chapter 11) of products that were suspected to contain allergens (such as a baked good), found this type of error uncommon but more likely to occur with smaller companies (a few products tested for milk or egg had trace amounts). Among 120 products that did not mention peanuts on the label, however, none had detectable peanut.

Do I need to call the manufacturers of every product to ask whether their food could be contaminated with an allergen?
It is difficult to recommend this degree of burdensome checking. As indicated above, the risks are generally low, and larger manufacturers (General Mills, Kraft, and so on) can generally be trusted. Caution about smaller companies, especially those making baked goods, may be advisable.

What do I do if I have an allergic reaction to a product and I do not know why?
If possible, keep the package, and then call the company and your allergist. You may have discovered a problem, such as an unintentional contamination with an allergen that could lead to a recall, or you may have an allergy to an ingredient you did not know about. You can contact the FDA's Center for Food Safety and Applied Nutrition (CFSAN) Adverse Event Reporting System by phone at 1-888-SAFEFOOD (1-888-723-3366) or online at www.fda.gov /AboutFDA/CentersOffices/OfficeofFoods/CFSAN/ContactCFSAN/.

What should I know about labeling laws in other countries?
Labeling laws vary among countries (and some have none). Many nations have laws that include more than just the major eight foods currently covered by US laws. Table 6.1 summarizes allergens covered by various countries, but of course these are subject to change. Research ahead of your trip to understand the laws where you are traveling.

Table 6.1. Allergens Covered by Labeling Laws in Different Countries

Country	Allergen
Australia and New Zealand	Milk, egg, peanut, wheat, gluten, crustacean shellfish, fish, soy, tree nuts, sesame
Canada	Milk, egg, peanut, wheat, gluten, crustacean shellfish, fish, soy, tree nuts, sesame, mustard, mollusks
European Union	Milk, egg, peanut, wheat, gluten, crustacean shellfish, fish, soy, tree nuts, sesame, mustard, mollusks, celery, lupine
Japan	Milk, egg, peanut, wheat, shrimp, crab, buckwheat
Korea	Milk, egg, peanut, wheat, shrimp, crab, buckwheat, fish, soy, peach, pork, tomato
United States	Milk, egg, peanut, wheat, crustacean shellfish, fish, soy, tree nuts (sesame starting January 2023)

How would I know if a mistake had been made in a food label?

Rarely, a food label will have an error, or a food allergen will have been added by mistake without labeling. Such foods, when identified, are recalled. You can get on a mailing list regarding food recalls for allergen-labeling errors at www.foodallergy.org/living-food-allergies/food-allergy-essentials/allergy -alerts.

Restaurants

Do restaurants know what to do for a person with food allergies?

Some may, but you should make no assumptions. Always discuss your allergy carefully with restaurant personnel.

Will the menu direct me to safe foods?

Some may, but you should never depend on a menu description to identify a safe meal. It is always possible that different ingredients are used than listed, that the list does not include all ingredients, or that the dish has unintended ingredients. Sometimes a food has been prepared ahead of your ordering it, or may have ingredients the people in the restaurant do not know about, so always discuss this possibility as well.

What types of mistakes can happen at a restaurant?
The food could have unintended ingredients, hidden or secret ingredients, or an allergen from cross-contact during preparation.

What are examples of hidden ingredients?
- A sauce thickened with peanut flour
- Fish used in a dressing
- Milk used in sauces
- Peanut butter used to seal the ends of an egg roll
- Nuts used in a dressing

How can I alert the restaurant personnel to my allergy?
The best action is to clearly identify that you have an allergy, not just a preference or distaste for a food. Explain that you could get sick if you ate even a small amount of the food you are avoiding. Provide some examples of what can be done wrong that would lead to a problem, as discussed below. Ask to speak with the person responsible for making your meal.

With whom should I communicate my needs at a restaurant?
You will usually begin a discussion with a server or manager. Suggest that you would like to speak with whomever is involved with preparing or overseeing the preparation of your meal. Providing some written description of your allergy—for example, a "chef card"—may help to emphasize your needs.

Where can I get "chef cards" for restaurant dining?
Examples are available at: https://www.foodallergy.org/resources/food -allergy-chef-cards.

Are certain types of restaurants off limits?
Some restaurants may be extremely poor choices, where the risks are too high (depending on the specific allergies). For example, a seafood restaurant is a poor choice for people with fish or shellfish allergies. Asian restaurants, bakeries, and ice cream shops can be a challenge for people with peanut or tree nut allergies. It is not always good enough to ask an ice

cream shop to wash the scoop because they may have already contaminated otherwise safe flavors when dipping from container to container. Self-serve buffets can be a challenge since food is often cross-contacted by the patrons. However, it may be possible to get a safe meal in any of these situations if the staff is understanding and accommodating and if you direct them appropriately.

What are some common pitfalls for people with food allergies eating in restaurants?

- Not explaining clearly that the problem is a true allergy (leading to a poor response)
- The staff making incorrect assumptions, for example, believing that removing an allergen from a finished dish is sufficient
- The staff not realizing an ingredient has allergens in it (such as milk in butter and egg in mayonnaise)
- Not considering cross-contact during food preparation (shared blenders, fryers, grills, serving utensils, etc.)
- The staff assuming they know the ingredients of a finished food
- Not considering the ingredients of all components of a meal (garnish, sauces)
- Not having medications (always carry your emergency medications)

What are some suggestions to help the restaurant staff provide a safe meal?

Be clear that you have a food allergy, that a small amount of the wrong food could send you to an emergency room or be life-threatening. Consider using chef cards that name your allergies and provide hints about allergen avoidance in restaurants. Ask to speak with people who are in charge, especially those who are responsible for the meal preparation, and provide some education as you make your requests by giving some concrete examples. Be specific. My studies on restaurant staff's knowledge showed that sometimes they make assumptions about food allergies that are incorrect (such as thinking that fryer heat destroys allergens).

What can I say to inform restaurant staff about preparing a safe meal?

Consider these examples:

- I am allergic to milk, and any bit of milk or milk products can make me very sick. I want a hamburger, no bun, steamed broccoli, and a baked potato. Please check if the hamburger has any fillers, because they could have milk. I want it cooked on foil on the grill to avoid getting cheese on it from a prior cheeseburger. If the potato or the vegetable looks dry, that is okay, but do not put butter on it!

- I am allergic to nuts, and any amount can make me sick. I want the salad without nuts. You cannot just pick the nuts off a premade salad. It has to be made from scratch. And if you chop nuts on a chopping board and then chop my lettuce, the lettuce can have nuts on it and make me sick. I will have the vinaigrette dressing if you can tell me the ingredients, because sometimes they flavor that with nuts. Otherwise, just bring me the oil and the vinegar.
- I am allergic to fish. I know I am just ordering French fries, but if you fry fish in the same oil, I could get sick.
- I am having the turkey sandwich, but I am extremely allergic to milk. Sometimes they flavor turkey with milk, so can you check that? Can I see the package ingredient label for the bread? I will skip it if it has milk. Also, if you slice the turkey on a slicer with cheese, I could get sick. Don't put any dressing on it because that often has milk. I will take ketchup.

What should I do if I think restaurant personnel are not understanding my allergy?
Leave.

What should I do if I get a meal that seems to have my allergen in it?
Hold the meal and ask to see the manager and chef. Sending a meal back could lead to more mistakes (such as having them remove the shrimp and re-serve the same pasta). If you are not comfortable, do not take a chance.

What are some options for going to restaurants with children who have food allergies?
One option is to bring along a safe meal that is similar to what the restaurant serves and explain the situation. It may be helpful to scout out a restaurant without your child first, to discuss what meals they may be able to make safely. Explain that you could become a frequent guest if they can accommodate your needs.

Social Outings and Family Gatherings

What are some concerns to consider when eating at other people's homes?

Family, friends, and acquaintances are usually not managing their homes day to day with concerns about food allergies. Well-intentioned hosts may not appreciate how to create a safe meal. Large, complex, multi-ingredient meals are associated with various social holidays, such as Christmas and Thanksgiving, as well as with milestone celebrations.

What should be done to obtain safe holiday meals away from home?

Speak with your hosts well in advance. Offer solutions, such as preparing simple, safe meals or bringing safe potluck contributions. Discuss your allergies as you would with a restaurant. Offer to help with meal preparation. When it is time for the meal, watch young, food-allergic children closely to be sure that they do not take unsafe foods from serving dishes or bowls with treats.

How should I arrange play dates for children with food allergies?

When introducing young children to friends' homes early on, explain your child's allergies and offer to stay for part of the time to explain about emergency medications. Bring safe snacks and discuss alternatives for snack times, or avoid snacks altogether. Be sure that your child, the friends, and supervising adults understand that the playdate should be stress-free so long as safe food is eaten, and that it should be easy to ensure that this happens. Children without food allergies are often interested in trying the "safe snacks."

Can a child with food allergy go trick-or-treating on Halloween?

Yes, but with planning ahead of time. It must be made clear that your child is not to eat any of the treats while out. Provide some safe snacks to bring along. Depending on the child's specific allergies, it may be possible to pick out safe foods based on ingredient labels once you are back home. Alternatively, arrange in advance to trade the bounty for safe treats or activities. For younger children, a few friends could be preselected who have or are provided with some safe treats that can be eaten right away. Never take chances on unlabeled treats!

School

What are the main concerns for going to school with food allergies?
The three main concerns are to (1) avoid eating a food allergen; (2) have a plan in place to treat an allergic reaction, especially anaphylaxis; and (3) learn and do everything that the other children are doing except for eating the avoided food.

How do I approach a school about managing my child's food allergies?
Discuss your child's food allergies well in advance. Begin by asking whether the school has other children with food allergies and what the school does to promote safety. I suggest this approach over presenting a large list of "requirements" that the school might view as overwhelming. Determine who coordinates food allergy management for the school. This is usually a school nurse, if there is one. Provide the school with the required documentation about the allergy from your doctor, and complete any forms that the school requires in advance. Work with your school, doctor, and child to develop a plan. Ensure that the management plan is communicated with all the individuals who will be supervising your child, including specialty teachers, such as for art, as well as substitute teachers. Discuss how safe meals and snacks will be obtained. Discuss how the emergency plans will be implemented, practiced, and extended to activities outside the school day, such as field trips, special events, and activities before or after school.

How does school food allergy management differ for various age groups?
The youngest preschool children are more apt to get into trouble by placing unsafe food—and almost anything else—in their mouths without concern. These children require strict supervision. Older children may understand not to share foods and can better self-manage. Teenagers should be able to self-manage, including recognizing and treating reactions, but this is also an age group that increases risk-taking, and you may not be able to depend on them to self-medicate with epinephrine. Supervision and avoidance strategies change according to age, developmental capabilities, and school resources. I discuss a child's age-related responsibilities later in this chapter.

Is it better to homeschool a child with food allergies to keep him or her safe?

Homeschooling is a fine choice if there is intrinsic interest in this educational approach, but it should not be necessary to homeschool a child solely because of a food allergy.

Are there any guidelines for managing food allergies in schools?

Yes. Although there are various state-initiated guidelines, the US Centers for Disease Control and Prevention worked with various experts (including me) and stakeholders to create a document titled "Voluntary Guidelines for Managing Food Allergies in Schools and Early Care and Education Programs." The report can be downloaded for free at www.cdc.gov/HealthyYouth /foodallergies/pdf/13_243135_A_Food_Allergy_Web_508.pdf. This terrific resource provides comprehensive advice.

What are the responsibilities of families sending their food-allergic children to school?

Review the checklist shown below:

CHECKLIST FOR FAMILIES:
GOING TO SCHOOL WITH FOOD ALLERGY

☐ Notify the school of your child's allergies.

☐ Work with the school team to develop a plan that accommodates the child's needs throughout the school, including in the classroom, in the cafeteria, in after-care programs, during school-sponsored activities, and on the school bus.

☐ Fill out a food allergy action plan (also called an allergy and anaphylaxis action plan, food allergy and anaphylaxis emergency plan, and so forth), and ensure that everyone on the school team has a copy.

☐ Provide written medical documentation, instructions, and medications as directed by a physician, using the food allergy action plan as a guide. Include a photo of your child on the written form.

☐ Provide properly labeled medications, and replace medications after use or upon expiration.

☐ Educate your child in food allergy self-management:
  • safe and unsafe foods
  • strategies for avoiding exposure to unsafe foods
  • symptoms of allergic reactions
  • how and when to tell an adult if having an allergy-related problem
  • how to read food labels (age appropriate)
☐ Review policies and procedures with the school staff, your child's physician, and your child (if age appropriate) after a reaction has occurred.
☐ Provide emergency contact information.
☐ Encourage your child to wear medical identification jewelry.

What are the responsibilities of the school for managing a child's food allergies?

A school's responsibilities may be summarized as follows:

• Be knowledgeable about and follow applicable federal laws, including the Americans with Disabilities Act, Section 504, and any state laws or district policies that apply.
• Review the health records submitted by parents and physicians.
• Include food-allergic students in school activities. Students should not be excluded from school activities based solely on their food allergies.
• Identify a core team of, but not limited to, school nurse, teacher, principal, school food service and nutrition manager, and counselor (if available) to work with parents and the student (age appropriate) to establish a prevention plan. Changes to the prevention plan to promote food allergy management should be made with core team participation.
• Make sure all staff who interact with the student understand food allergy, can recognize symptoms, know what to do in an emergency, and work with other school staff to eliminate the use of food allergens in the allergic student's meals, educational tools, arts and crafts projects, and incentives.
• Practice the food allergy action plans before an allergic reaction occurs to ensure the efficiency/effectiveness of the plans.
• Coordinate with the school nurse to ensure that medications are appropriately stored, and be sure to make available an emergency kit that

contains a physician's standing order for epinephrine. In states where regulations permit, medications are kept in an easily accessible, secure location central to designated school personnel, not in locked cupboards or drawers.

- Students should be allowed to carry their own epinephrine, if age appropriate, after approval from the student's physician or clinic, parent, and school nurse, as allowed by state or local regulations. See below for more information on this decision.
- Designate school personnel who are properly trained to administer medications in accordance with the state nursing and Good Samaritan laws governing the administration of emergency medications.
- Be prepared to handle a reaction, and ensure that a staff member who is properly trained to administer medications is available during the school day regardless of time or location.
- Review policies and prevention plans with core team members, parents or guardians, the student (age appropriate), and the physician after a reaction has occurred.
- Work with the district transportation administrator to make sure that school bus driver training includes symptom awareness and what to do if a reaction occurs.
- Recommend that all buses have communication devices in case of an emergency.
- Enforce a "no eating" policy on school buses, with exceptions made only to accommodate special needs under federal or similar laws, or school district policy.
- Discuss appropriate management of food allergy with student families.
- Discuss field trips with the families of food-allergic children to decide appropriate strategies for managing the allergies.
- Follow federal, state, and district laws and regulations regarding sharing medical information about the student.
- Take seriously any threats against and harassment or bullying of an allergic child (see chapter 7 for more on bullying).

What are the students' responsibilities for managing food allergies in school?

The students' responsibilities will vary by age and developmental level but may be summarized as follows:

- Should not trade food with others
- Should not eat anything with unknown ingredients or known to contain any allergen
- Should be proactive in the care and management of their food allergies and reactions based on their developmental level
- Should notify an adult immediately if they eat something they believe may contain the food to which they are allergic

What role does handwashing play in food allergen avoidance?

It is presumed that handwashing would reduce finger-to-mouth transfer of allergens should the child with food allergies touch an allergen. It is presumed that classmates' handwashing after meals would reduce spread of food allergens to materials that are shared by classmates. But these strategies have not really been tested. Based on what is known about the amounts of foods that might trigger reactions and the low risk of severe reactions from skin exposure, one might expect that handwashing would play a minor role in protecting children with food allergies compared to policies such as not sharing food. The relative benefits may also be influenced by the age of the children, since younger children may be more apt to put fingers or toys in their mouths.

Do antibacterial gels and foams remove allergens from hands?

No, just germs. To get allergens off dirty hands requires soap and water or wet wipes.

Do schools or classrooms need to exclude (ban) food allergens?

Banning a food from a specific classroom or a school is one option that is sometimes undertaken to reduce risk. Most often, the ban is applied to peanut and tree nuts. Classroom bans are more common than school-wide ones and are more often aimed at children who are too young to self-monitor. No studies prove that this is an effective strategy, but it is assumed to reduce the risk. One study focusing on peanut suggested that regarding rate of administration of epinephrine, various bans were not effective but peanut-free tables were (see Bartnikas et al. in chapter 11). Even so, it remains crucial to enforce the additional strategies listed above to ensure safety. Bans can lead to a false sense of security ("I can share food since nothing has peanut") and to allergic reactions from these false assumptions. Personal issues and the age of the child may come into play in decision-making. For example, it may be sensible to "ban" powdery, messy, cheese-puff-type snacks from a kindergarten room when one student has a severe milk allergy.

What type of cleaning needs to be done to keep eating areas safe for children with food allergies?

No special chemicals are needed. Soap and water or a wet wipe are typically sufficient to remove allergens. There would need to be some type of physical motion to wipe off the surfaces, not just spreading the residue around, even if soap is used.

Can cafeterias provide safe meals for children with food allergies?

Yes, but they must understand how to do so. Talk to your school beforehand to ensure they can successfully avoid the allergens (understand cross-contact, label reading, etc.). Another option is to provide a bagged lunch and snack.

What are some safe food alternatives for children with food allergies in school?

Foods used for craft projects, science experiments, celebrations, and snacks can be substituted. Watch out for unexpected food exposure, such as egg white used to smooth finger paint or wheat in modeling clays. If foods must be used, consider alternatives such as rice milk for cow's milk. Nonfood treats can be substituted as rewards or for celebrations, for example, birthday pencils or other trinkets. Have safe, nonperishable snacks available for spontaneous celebrations. Talk to the school personnel to make sure that they communicate any special events in advance so that everyone is aware of any issues about food allergy and can address them ahead of time.

What are some alternatives for school celebrations that involve food?

The teacher might instead have a fun activity, such as watching a movie; reading a special book; handing out trinkets, such as birthday pencils, small stuffed animals, or other toys; or adding time to recess instead of having a food celebration. Celebrations could include games with prizes or an arts and crafts project.

How should snack times be managed for children with food allergies?

There are several ways. The responsible adults might ensure that any snack is safe for the entire class; there might be substitute snacks for those with food allergies; or snacks might be limited, with alternative nonfood options for celebrations, such as a celebratory game or toy.

How should lunch and mealtimes be managed for children with food allergies?

It depends on the child's age. Younger children will need more supervision. If there is no allergen-safe table, more supervision to prevent sharing may be needed. The allergic child might be seated toward a table's end and near a supervising adult. It is generally good practice to limit mealtimes to locations designated for them when possible, rather than having young children carry snacks or food throughout play areas, where the allergic child might take them. If the meal is eaten at a table that can be cleaned afterward and then used for any other activities, there is less chance that foods of danger to the young child will be left in reach. I am not in favor of having a child sit alone or separated. If there is a medical need to keep the child away from others eating the allergen, which would be quite unusual, then options such as inviting some friends who are eating safe foods to eat with the child who has allergies is an option. Older children who are not likely to take unsafe foods from others would usually require much less supervision or concern.

Do we need an allergen-free table or cafeteria?

I prefer the term "allergen-safe" when designating a table or cafeteria as a place where peanuts or nuts are not allowed. Whether you believe your child needs this type of accommodation would require consideration of your child's age and ability to understand not taking another child's food, as well as of particular circumstances of the allergy and school setting described previously. My bias is that most children with food allergies who know not to take another's food should not need special seating arrangements. The options should be discussed with your allergist and school. A 2021 guideline on managing food allergy in schools and childcare centers (see Waserman et al. in chapter 11) deterred the use of allergen bans except in special circumstances, as previously discussed.

Why do you prefer the term "allergen-safe" rather than "allergen-free"?

This is to avoid the notion that food sharing would be acceptable if allergens were banned. In reality, people who are not living with food allergies on a daily basis may not be sending "safe" foods to school. There could be a false sense of security. I am aware of reactions in "peanut-free" settings because of this circumstance.

How should preschool time and afterschool activities and sports be managed for children with food allergies?

Ensure that all of the adults who are supervising a child with food allergies are aware of the allergies. Otherwise, unsafe foods might be offered, reactions unnoticed, and emergency plans not arranged properly.

Does a child with food allergies need a paraprofessional to maintain safety in the school setting?

A paraprofessional is an individual assigned to provide individualized attention to a child, in this case to assist the child in avoiding the food and recognizing or initiating treatment of an allergic reaction. The decision to request or grant this level of service is individualized according to the child, the allergies, and the school circumstances. In my experience, the need for this is exceptional because there are many options for successful avoidance.

What should be done about bus transportation for children with food allergies?

Ideally, the bus driver would be able to take responsibility for a child's food allergy just as a teacher does. Local regulations, however, may prevent the driver from taking on the full responsibilities of an emergency action plan. Good Samaritan laws would still apply in an emergency.

What are the key issues to address regarding bus transportation for a child with food allergies?

- Ensure that the driver is informed about your child's allergies, symptoms, and requirements for treatment in the event of an allergic reaction.
- Request no eating on the bus.
- Have younger children with food allergies sit at the front of the bus, under closer supervision of the driver.
- Insist that the driver have a communication device, such as a cell phone, and discuss emergency procedures, such as calling 911 and providing the necessary details in the event of an emergency on the bus (this would include not only allergy but also any other general emergencies, such as a bus accident, or medical emergencies, such as seizures or injuries).

Should there be epinephrine on the bus?

Ideally, self-injectable epinephrine would be on board, but sometimes circumstances and regulations prevent this option. The child may be allowed to self-carry, but depending on the child, self-injecting is not usually reasonable. See additional discussion on these topics later in this chapter.

What can be done to reduce the risk of a food-allergic reaction on the bus?

The risk of having an allergic reaction on the school bus is minimized by ensuring the student has a safe meal and no symptoms prior to boarding. The most serious error I have seen was a school placing a child on a bus during an allergic reaction under the misguided notion that the child would best be managed by the parent upon arrival at home. The degree of concern and special accommodations might vary according to your child's age, developmental ability, and specific allergies, but most children with food allergies are able to ride the school bus safely with the minimal accommodations described above. Concerns about significant reactions from residual, invisible food proteins on seats are not typically warranted, but a seat could be cleaned with a wet wipe if needed for a young child.

How should field trips be managed for children with food allergies?

Remind the school about extending food allergy management to activities outside the school building. Parents should be informed about field trips in advance. Decisions may need to be made about avoiding high-risk activities, for example, touring a peanut factory for a child with peanut allergy. Safe meals would need to be arranged in advance, such as a bagged lunch, and an adult who is able to recognize and treat allergic reactions should be available.

What emergency plans should be in place in the event of an allergic reaction at school?

Individuals supervising your child should be educated about the allergy, recognition of symptoms, and how to activate an emergency response, such as promptly giving epinephrine. In some cases, this would mean that the supervising adult provides treatment, but in most cases, it means alerting the on-site health care professional or that person's delegate. The emergency plan typically includes providing medications according to symptoms, activating emergency services by calling 911, and then informing parents.

Although a written plan that authorizes treatment is essential, everyone involved should be familiar with the actions they should be taking. They should not need to read the plan or begin to learn how to use an epinephrine autoinjector at the time of an emergency—they should have rehearsed how to do what they need to do in advance!

Who is responsible for the emergency plans in a school?

The school nurse is typically responsible for the details of the emergency plans and for educating others about the allergy and treatment response, including when and how to use epinephrine. Otherwise, it may be necessary to work through school administration.

What are the differences in management for schools with and without a school nurse?

When there is no on-site school nurse, delegates would be required to understand how to recognize and manage food allergies. Even with a nurse, this is good policy because others in the school are able to provide backup. Often, the principal and vice principal take primary responsibility, but additional teachers may be part of the management team. When there is an on-site school nurse, it is often preferable to alert that person to manage an allergic reaction. There would typically not be much time lost in alerting a school nurse through an intercom system, but having backup delegates available in case of delay is prudent.

Does each child in a school require his or her own emergency plan and medications?

Every child with a food allergy should have their own written emergency plan. New laws allow a general prescription of and administration of epinephrine to children who do not have a prior anaphylaxis diagnosis or emergency plan. Most states have adopted stock epinephrine laws, which allow for schools to keep epinephrine on hand for use in persons without a prior known allergy, and an increasing number of states require it. For some schools this may also mean that each child with an emergency plan for their food allergies need not be required to supply an autoinjector for personal use. You can check the law in your state at www.foodallergy.org/our-initiatives/advocacy/food-allergy-issues/school-access-epinephrine.

What key points should be addressed for emergency management of an allergic reaction in school?

- There should be a written action plan that the supervising adults are familiar with.
- There should be a procedure in place for activation of the plan in the event of an emergency, such as a strategy to promptly inform the nurse or delegate.
- Procedures for obtaining and administering emergency medications should be well known and rehearsed.
- Procedures for activating emergency services and communicating with parents should be rehearsed.
- Emergency plans should be considered in the context of special circumstances, such as field trips, special activities, and emergencies such as a lockdown.

Where should epinephrine be stored?

Ideally, in a widely known, unlocked location with prompt access. Depending on the school's physical layout, this may entail a location in or near a cafeteria, in the administration's office, or in the nursing office.

How many doses of epinephrine should be available?

At least two doses should be accessible.

Should a student carry emergency medications?

When the student is capable of self-carrying and self-treatment, and local guidelines allow it, this is a reasonable approach, especially if the medication would otherwise not be accessible within a few minutes.

How does one know when a student is capable of carrying emergency medications?

Below are some considerations for carrying emergency medications.

For students

- They express a desire to carry and self-administer epinephrine.
- They are deemed of appropriate age, maturity, or developmental level.
- They can identify signs and symptoms of anaphylaxis.
- They can demonstrate knowledge of proper medication use in response to signs and symptoms.

- They demonstrate correct technique in administering epinephrine (with a trainer).
- They are willing to comply with school's rules about use of medicine at school, for example:
  - keeping the autoinjector of epinephrine with them at all times
  - immediately notifying a responsible adult (teacher, nurse, coach, playground assistant) when autoinjectable epinephrine is used
  - not sharing medication with other students or leaving it unattended
  - not using autoinjectable epinephrine for any other use than what is intended

For parents or guardians
- They desire for the student to self-carry and self-administer.
- They are aware of school medication policies and parental responsibilities.
- They are committed to making sure students have the needed medication with them, medications are refilled when needed, backup medications are provided, and medication use at school is monitored through collaborative effort between the parent or guardian and the school team.

How does one know when a student is capable of self-treating an allergic reaction?

Most children over about age 7 can physically activate a self-injector, but no child should be depended on to do so in an emergency. If your school allows your child to self-carry, be sure to emphasize that this situation does not mitigate the need for an adult to take full responsibility for administering the medication in the event of an emergency. A survey of pediatric allergists suggested that they usually expect some transfer of responsibility by ages 12 to 14 years. There is no "correct" age for all children, however.

Some children may not be considered responsible enough to be carrying their medications because they tend to play with the medications and could injure themselves or another child. Other children may be responsible, but some of the children around them may not be and could take the medication if not supervised well enough, possibly risking injury. The answer also depends on a child's ability to understand the illness and appropriate treatment in the event of a reaction.

What is a Section 504 plan with regard to food allergy?

There is a public law (Section 504) that prohibits discrimination in education for any type of disability. The law applies to programs that receive federal funds and was developed for children with educational disabilities as well as vision and hearing impairment. The same law has been applied for children with other medical conditions, including allergies. Section 504 can be set up to require the school to have a plan that makes it safe for your child to attend the school and learn effectively as well as ensures that an emergency plan is in place; the plan can specify substitutions so that your child can participate in various activities with others.

Do I need a Section 504 plan to keep my child safe?

Most often, schools follow simple procedures and guidelines to ensure safety for children with food allergies without the need to invoke an individual Section 504 plan. Most of my patients do not develop Section 504 plans because they are able to obtain the needed accommodations for their child by discussing these needs with the administration and school nurse, providing a written emergency action plan that describes the allergy, and supplying the medications to treat a reaction. If you are having trouble with the school providing a safe environment, however, and the school receives federal funds, it is possible to set up a Section 504 plan to achieve the needed goals. The type of plan that is more directed to health issues, however, is the individualized health care plan.

What is an individualized health care plan?

A student's individualized health care plan, or IHCP, is typically developed by the school nurse in collaboration with the family, the child's physician, and other school personnel. The plan may include an emergency action plan that describes the allergy, symptoms, and treatments, as well as the means to avoid reactions, the roles of individuals in the child's care, and other aspects included in various state or national guidelines.

What issues arise for college students? What should students do in preparation?

All the points made about school management, and food allergy management in general, apply in college except that the person with food allergies has more independent responsibility and will need to take more control of avoidance and treatment issues. Discuss food allergy management well ahead of college decision time. I recommend discussing college issues with your allergist years in advance. Many times, families and the student become interested in performing additional definitive diagnostic tests, such as the oral food challenge, prior to the student embarking on these last years toward independence. It is crucial to make sure the young adult knows how to avoid food allergens and how to self-treat in the event of anaphylaxis. Reading this book should help! Once you have your college chosen, let the office of disability services know about your food allergy, and work with them to ensure proper accommodations.

Are there colleges that specialize in students with food allergies?

Some colleges may have more experience with students requiring special meals, but decisions about attending college should not be tied to food allergy. Most colleges are now capable of providing the necessary accommodations.

What living conditions at college should be addressed with regard to food allergy?

Meeting with food service personnel is important and might be arranged during preadmission visits. Personal preferences (living in a dormitory and having a meal plan versus living in housing with a kitchen and cooking for oneself) should be discussed. Roommates might be viewed as a liability if there is a shared kitchen because of cross-contact of allergens. But having roommates has significant advantages for socialization and can mean having others to watch out for the person with an allergy in the event of a reaction. Many schools have become significantly more allergy aware in the past several years, and programs are available to colleges regarding food allergen safety (for example, from www.foodallergy.org).

Camp

What are some unique issues for staying safe with food allergies while at camp?

All the same concerns for management in school apply to camps, as well as a few additional concerns:

- Supervising individuals may be young and inexperienced
- Activities may bring the child into remote areas (hikes)
- Attending overnight camps requires extensive provision of safe meals

Can a child with food allergies attend overnight camp?
Yes, so long as the concerns about allergen avoidance and recognition and treatment of an allergic reaction can be accommodated.

What are some ways to maintain safety in summer camps for children with food allergies?
- Discuss your child's food allergy well in advance, prior to committing to the experience.
- Ask what the camp has done in the past to manage children with food allergies.
- Discuss approaches that were successful at school and how they can be applied to the camp experience.
- Speak with food service personnel and camp health services.
- Review the camp's approaches to daily activities that affect food allergy management.

Work

What are some unique concerns in the workplace for individuals with food allergy?
Coworkers may be less knowledgeable or understanding about food allergies. It may be difficult to maintain safe communal food areas. For example, a coffee maker might be used to make nut-flavored coffee, causing risks for an individual with nut allergies. Food storage or preparation areas might contain allergens. Thus the allergic individual may need to take extra care in storing and preparing safe foods.

What types of food allergies are unique to the workplace?
Occupational food allergies most often develop in manufacturing plants or bakeries. A person with baker's asthma can eat wheat but develop asthma symptoms when inhaling powdery flour during food preparation. Other airborne food proteins used in or caused by manufacturing include powdered milk and eggs, fish, and shellfish. Persistent, itchy rashes from direct skin contact with food proteins can also occur.

What foods might cause skin reactions in the workplace?
For food handlers and manufacturers, the list of skin allergens and irritants is long. Some of the more common triggers are fruits, garlic, onion, raw fish, raw meat, raw shellfish, seeds, spices, and vegetables. Almost every food has caused some form of allergy for handlers in the workplace.

What are some tips to make the workplace safe for people with food allergies?
In food manufacturing settings, workers who are sensitive to the foods being worked with might wear goggles, masks, and gloves. Sometimes, occupational allergy to foods cannot be easily overcome, and an alternative job must be sought.

For nonindustrial settings, an individual with food allergy must take care in food storage and preparation, and must be cautious about ingesting foods from others who may not understand details about food allergen avoidance. For example, a well-meaning coworker might make "nut-free" cookies but not understand the trace contamination introduced while preparing the food at home. Applying the "rules" about allergen avoidance described previously will promote safety in the workplace.

Travel

What should I do to prepare for traveling safely with food allergies?
Avoiding an allergen during travel and vacation is similar to avoiding it in restaurants, except there may be additional concerns, such as language barriers. Planning ahead is crucial to avoid mishaps. There are fewer options without the ability to prepare meals at home, so it may be helpful to consider lodging that offers a kitchenette. Call ahead to hotels and restaurants to discuss the allergy and ensure that there are safe options. Choose uncomplicated meals that are prepared simply to avoid cross-contact and hidden ingredients. Carry all medications and instructions. Be familiar with activating emergency services. Obtain location-specific allergy information (see chapter 11). Consider your destination's labeling laws (discussed earlier in this chapter).

How far from medical care can a person with food allergies be and still be safe?
Having a food allergy should not limit travel. Although it is ideal to be able to obtain advanced medical care quickly—for example, in less than 30 minutes—this may not be possible. If the travel is remote, ensuring that all foods are entirely safe is crucial.

How many epinephrine autoinjectors should I carry?
Typical instructions are to have two doses available at all times, so, depending on the circumstances of the trip and considering that it may not be easy to refill a used autoinjector, it might be wise to carry at least one or two extra doses. More doses may be warranted for prolonged travel in remote areas.

Are there preferred, safe travel destinations for persons with food allergies?
Some destinations may be easier to manage. For example, a trip to a country where communication is limited would be much more difficult than one to a country where you can communicate fluently. Call ahead to theme parks, because some are particularly allergy friendly. Disney has received awards for its approach to food allergies, for example. With enough preparation, you should be able to travel without being excessively limited by food allergies.

What are the main concerns about airplane travel with food allergies?
Airplane travel can provoke anxiety because of the isolation and distance from medical care. Persons with peanut allergies face the possibility of experiencing symptoms when many people in the cabin are opening powdery peanut snacks. The symptoms are usually mild. More severe symptoms are possible if the avoided food is eaten. Talk with your doctor about the potential risks as they apply to you or to your child's allergies and personal circumstances. Most of the time, the concerns would not warrant changing travel plans.

What are some strategies for traveling safely on airplanes with food allergy?
- Check the airline's website for details about the snacks and other food served on board flights. Also check the website www.foodallergy.org for updates on airline policies.

- Notify the airline about the allergy.
- Call ahead to the airline to discuss any special concerns.
- Obtain a note from your doctor that indicates permission to carry medications and other supplies and foods because of the allergy (see chapter 11 for an example).
- Carry your medications and an emergency action plan that describes the allergy.
- Keep your medication in its original packaging, which includes prescription labels.
- Bring safe snacks and foods (do not trust the airline meals).
- Consider taking an earlier flight, when allergenic snacks may not be served.
- For young children with food allergies, check for leftover food on tray tables, in seat pockets, and in the seats, including cracks between seat cushions. Consider using a wet wipe on the seating and tray surfaces.

What are the primary concerns about travel on cruise ships with food allergies?

Similar to airplane travel, cruises present isolation from advanced medical care. Perhaps to a greater degree than other types of travel, there is dependence on others for providing safe foods. Therefore it is recommended to call ahead to discuss your individual circumstances and ensure that safe meals will be obtainable.

Dating and Relationships

Is it possible to have an allergic reaction from kissing?

Yes. About 10% of adults with food allergies describe having had such reactions, which are usually mild. They occur because residual protein in the saliva can be ingested through passionate kissing. An innocent kiss on the cheek is not likely to result in a significant reaction; more typically, no symptoms are observed, or at most a localized swelling occurs.

How can I reduce the risk of an allergic reaction from kissing?

One study examined the time course of finding peanut protein in the saliva of people who ate an entire peanut butter sandwich (see Maloney et al. in chapter 11). The amount of protein declined rapidly in the hours after eating the sandwich. Brushing teeth, rinsing the mouth, and chewing gum all significantly reduced the amount of residual protein to levels not likely to cause severe reactions, but there was some residual protein. The most effective strategy was to allow about four hours to pass and to have had a peanut-free meal; in that situation, we could not detect the peanut protein. This type of testing has not been tried with other foods, and presumably there is potential for solid bits of allergen—for example, a tiny nut crumb—to dislodge from between teeth and cause a reaction in a partner. Therefore the safest bet is to have an intimate partner avoid the allergen or at least eat a safe meal before passionate kissing.

Is it possible to have an allergic reaction from intercourse?

It is theoretically possible for food allergens to enter seminal fluid and potentially cause reactions in a sensitive partner. However, this theory has not been proven. There are rare case reports where allergic reactions to seminal fluids were attributed to foods or medications, but more often these reactions are due to actual allergy to the components of sperm and seminal fluids. Nonetheless, safety about kissing may apply to intercourse as well.

What are some tips to maintain safety for dating and relationships when there is food allergy?

It is particularly important to ensure that a partner is aware of the allergy so that precautions can be taken. Playing kissing games or indiscriminate intimacy with strangers or persons who are not aware of the allergy could have bad consequences for people with food allergies. Teenagers in particular should be aware of this concern.

Age-Related Responsibilities

How do food allergy management responsibilities change with age?

As children get older, they can take increasing responsibility for allergen avoidance and treatment of any reactions. The exact ages for transferring various responsibilities depend on personal factors, the family's comfort, and individual developmental factors. Talk to your child, doctor, teachers, and others to best understand what responsibilities should gradually be transferred.

How do I determine whether my child can take on more responsibility for managing food allergies?

Observe your child in various situations to gauge readiness for increasing responsibility. Consider involving others, for example, to find out if your child will accept food from a stranger.

How do I encourage my child to become more independent with managing food allergies?

Reward successes and be positive about progress, even if it seems that failures are preventing a transition to independence. The process should be consistent and gradual so that a teenager, based on years of experience, feels comfortable managing the allergies appropriately and experiences no awkwardness telling others about them.

What food allergy management responsibilities might be expected of a toddler?

Very few. This is a time to begin education. Introduce the concept of there being safe and unsafe foods. Try to use terms that are clear. For example, for a child with milk allergy, it is better practice to refer to "John's soy drink" rather than "John's special milk" to avoid misunderstandings about cow's milk versus soy "milk."

What food allergy management responsibilities might be expected of a preschool child?

At this age, the child should be taught that certain adults know what foods are safe. "Only Mom, Dad, Aunt Susie, and Grandma know what food you can eat safely. If you take food from other people, you could get sick." Although your child may know which foods to avoid, you should emphasize not accepting foods from people who are not "approved" by you. A preschooler may not be depended on to follow this rule and may grab foods, so constant supervision is needed.

What food allergy management responsibilities might be expected of a 5-to-6-year-old?

For this age group, continue to emphasize not taking foods unless approved by a responsible adult, and expect your child to demonstrate this. Some children begin to understand the role of emergency medications at this age, but they are not usually ready to carry them responsibly. They should be taught to report symptoms to an adult. This is a good age for children to be taught how to comfortably inform others about their allergy.

What food allergy management responsibilities might be expected of a 7-to-10-year-old?

In this age group, children can partner with an adult to read ingredient labels, choose safe foods, and talk about their allergies in restaurants. A responsible adult still needs to oversee these actions and use this as a learning time. Some children in this age group might be trusted to carry medications but generally not to decide on when to use them.

What food allergy management responsibilities might be expected of a 10-to-12-year-old?

Under adult supervision, children in this age group should be capable of discussing their allergies with restaurant personnel and correctly choosing safe foods. If appropriate according to school regulations, they may carry medications responsibly and should understand when to use them, although they would not be depended on to do so.

What food allergy management responsibilities might be expected of a 13-to-18-year-old?

This is the age when children can take responsibility for obtaining safe meals and reporting and treating symptoms. This is also an age of risk-taking, however, so these responsibilities still require supervision. Teenagers should be frequently coached about their allergies and treatment. These issues are discussed further in chapter 4.

Special Exposure Risks

As a breastfeeding mother, do I need to avoid eating foods my child is allergic to?

It depends, and this situation should be discussed with your child's allergist. The amount of allergen found in breast milk is typically very low. It varies by individual and by how much was eaten. Allergy to foods in maternal breast milk has been linked to infants having flaring or eczema, mucous and blood in stools (proctocolitis), and, very rarely, anaphylaxis.

What dietary options do I have while breastfeeding my food-allergic child?

Options include strict avoidance, reduced ingestion, no change, or ingestion of specific forms of the food, for example, eggs or milk in bakery goods and not as whole milk or eggs. These considerations must be discussed with your or your child's doctor.

What factors might my allergist consider when deciding whether I should avoid eating the foods my child is allergic to while I'm still breastfeeding?

We do not know whether trace exposure to the allergen in breast milk speeds, hinders, or has no effect on a child's allergy recovery, so allergists primarily consider the risk of allergic reactions in the infant as well as nutritional and social factors for the mother.

If your child was perfectly fine on breast milk and had only mild symptoms when directly ingesting the food, you may not have to alter your diet, or you may be advised not to exceed specified amounts of ingestion. If your child had chronic symptoms while being breastfed, any sudden reactions to your breast milk after you ingested an allergen, or a severe reaction when ingesting the food directly, there is stronger reason for you to avoid the food in your own diet, or to dramatically reduce ingestion.

The type of food involved is another consideration. For example, it may be easier and more prudent to avoid peanuts, nuts, fish, or shellfish for an infant diagnosed with these severe allergies, but if your child has a mild milk allergy, reducing your cow's milk consumption, or ingesting only baked forms, may be reasonable. Always talk to your allergist, and be sure to address nutritional issues if you need to avoid certain foods.

If I accidentally ate an allergen, such as peanuts, how long will it be in my breast milk?

This has not been extensively studied. In one small study, about half of mothers had detectable peanut in their breast milk after eating peanuts. It was usually found within two hours of ingestion and typically gone by eight hours, as tested by intermittent pumping.

Do medications contain food allergens?

They may, although this is not a common concern. Reports of allergic reactions to food proteins in medications are actually quite rare. The ingredients of medications are typically disclosed in package inserts, although not in the same manner as on food labels. Ask your pharmacist and allergist. In some cases, a call to the manufacturer is needed. Most medication flavoring is artificial, but it is sensible to check. Coconut is a rare allergen, and coconut oil may have only trace proteins, but this is sometimes an ingredient in medications. Oils used in some medications are typically highly refined, and allergy risks are therefore minimal. Propofol, a type of injected anesthetic agent, has an ingredient derived from egg; there is no clear, documented risk for persons with egg allergy, but using an alternative can help avoid the theoretical risk. In all cases, discuss any concerns with your allergist.

Is lactose in medications a concern for those with milk allergy?

Pharmaceutical-grade lactose may sometimes contain trace residual milk proteins. You will need to ask your allergist if this is a concern. See chapter 1 for more information.

Do vaccines contain food allergens?

See chapter 1 for a discussion of food allergens in vaccines.

Do hospitals understand how to prepare safe meals for someone with food allergies?

They should, but do not assume so. Always check with the hospital personnel before eating meals (each one), and treat food services as you treat those serving you in a restaurant. See the discussion of ways to explain your allergy to those who prepare and serve your food earlier in this chapter.

Can blood transfusions trigger allergic reactions because of food allergy?

Theoretically, if a blood donor has eaten an allergen, it may appear in trace amounts in their bloodstream and be a problem for a recipient. When blood transfusions are processed, however, the liquid (serum) is washed away, so even if trace proteins had been in the blood donation, the amount left in the material that is transfused would be negligible. There have not been reports of reactions in this situation, although it may be reasonable for a donor providing a directed donation to a person with a food allergy to avoid the allergen for several hours prior to the donation. There is one report of a platelet donation causing a reaction in a child with peanut allergy (platelets are the blood-clotting component transfused without being separated from the serum). The report is not completely verified, but there may be a risk.

Delving Deeper

Eleven-year-old Andrew was diagnosed with a peanut allergy based on an allergic reaction at age 1 year. His family spent many years ensuring no exposure to peanut. Over time, they stopped going to restaurants and relatives' homes, and they did not take vacations because they were worried about allergens in places away from home, and they wanted to ask me about finding a dog that can "sniff out" peanuts. At the same time, Andrew wanted to know if he could eat foods that say "may contain" peanut.

Andrew's family had been told that he is "severely allergic" based on testing at age 3, but they had not had a discussion about threshold or severity of his allergy or about risks of ingestion compared to skin contact or smell. When I saw him at age 11 years, Andrew had tests that were convincing for peanut allergy, but he had no asthma, and no exposure to peanut except for a large serving that resulted in facial hives at age 1. I reviewed these relative risks (as described in this chapter) and how the family could manage Andrew's allergy in a way that could allow him to do everything that other children his age do, short of ingesting peanut. It is a lot of work, but by informing others, reading labels, speaking with restaurant personnel, and taking modest steps to prepare, Andrew would do well.

We conducted a quick contact test where I had Andrew hold a peanut, and showed that nothing happened. I explained that about half of people with peanut allergy might have mild or no symptoms from an amount of peanut equivalent to one kernel. We discussed and then undertook a graded oral food challenge (see chapter 3) to a small amount of peanut, which he tolerated. He did not begin to have symptoms until he ate the equivalent of two peanuts. Regarding the "peanut-sniffing dog," I explained that although there are positive testimonials about such animals, my allergist colleagues and I have reservations. The dogs are not able to accurately "approve" a safe meal. Since there are typically no significant risks of being near peanut so long as the person is not eating peanut, the dog's main capability of identifying peanut is not crucial to avoiding eating the allergen. Additionally, having a dog only for peanut allergy avoidance presents a social and emotional factor that may seem empowering or comforting, but could also result in a feeling of vulnerability that is greater than necessary or result in isolation that is not necessary. Finally, allowing such a dog into schools or on planes may result in allergen exposure to persons with a dog dander allergy.

Regarding the question about "may contain peanut" and advisory labeling in general, we discussed the relative risks. The literature about these risks is incomplete. Worldwide, two deaths have been reported regarding ignoring advisory labels for peanut. Based on various studies, roughly 5% to 10% of the products with warnings contain the allergen, usually in small amounts. Several studies suggest that people who ignore advisory labeling are at a risk of having reactions, but the rates are unclear (rates around 5% are noted in a few studies, but people who are most allergic may take fewer risks). Given the quality-of-life issues for Andrew, his high threshold of reaction to peanut, and lack of asthma, he, his parents, and I agreed that advisory labeling was not a significant risk for him.

CHAPTER 7

Maintaining Lifestyle and Quality of Life, Reducing Anxiety, and Keeping a Healthy Diet

Daily lifestyle issues are a major concern for people who are living with food allergies. In this chapter I explore emotional concerns and interpersonal relationships. I also explain nutritional management, including maintaining a healthy diet.

General Questions about Lifestyle and Quality of Life

In what ways might food allergy affect lifestyle and health?
Living with food allergies can be limiting in many ways. Social occasions and each meal and snack present potential obstacles. Obtaining foods becomes time consuming. The burden on individuals and families can become great. Social activities and vacationing can be affected. Anxiety may increase because of the constant diligence and fear associated with each meal. Nutritional concerns may arise if the diet is limited, posing additional health concerns. Overall, social, emotional, and general health may be affected.

What is "health-related quality of life" as it relates to food allergy?
The term "health-related quality of life" refers to the impact that a health condition, in this case food allergy, may have on three major aspects of overall health: physical, social, emotional, or psychological well-being. Many people with food allergies "look fine," so it is often hard for others

to understand the significant repercussions that living with a food allergy has on individuals and families.

Are there any simple ways to improve quality of life among people with food allergies?

One goal should be to ensure that the person with food allergies is able to do everything that people without food allergies do except for eating the food to which they are allergic. Achieving this goal may not always be simple. The first step is to identify whether there is a problem, and then to work with your health care professional to determine whether the trouble is

- related to concerns about food allergy or some other cause
- a reasonable or an excessive concern in relation to your allergies
- treatable through simple education or requires more elaborate interventions

How might I know if food allergy is causing more of an impact on quality of life than it should?

Take time to discuss living with food allergies with your health care professional, even if you feel that you have everything under control. Sometimes you may be doing something you feel is warranted, that does not significantly affect your lifestyle, but it could actually be unnecessarily limiting in comparison to how most people with food allergies live their lives.

For example, I was shocked to learn of a family who had their child with food allergies eat in a room away from the rest of the family just because they thought they needed to take this precaution. Other families might never go to a restaurant because of food allergies. These dramatic decisions are almost never necessary. Consider the list of concerns in table 7.1. If any of these apply to you or your child, discuss them with your allergist.

Could having an allergic reaction improve quality of life?

Yes. You would think that a food-allergic reaction would mostly increase anxiety, and it could, but a study looking at doctor-supervised feeding tests (oral food challenges) showed improvement in measurements of quality of life regardless of whether the test resulted in a reaction (see Franxman et al. in chapter 11). This could be because the person experiencing the reaction learned that (1) he or she is avoiding the food for a good reason or (2) the reaction symptoms were recognizable and manageable, countering anxiety about what a food-allergic reaction might entail.

Table 7.1. Checklist of Concerns to Discuss with Your Allergist

- ☐ Choosing a vacation is a problem
- ☐ Choosing a restaurant is a problem
- ☐ Participating in social activities with food is a problem
- ☐ Worrying a lot about allergic reactions
- ☐ Feeling sadness about food allergy
- ☐ Participating in school or work activities is a problem
- ☐ Feeling like it is too hard to manage food allergy
- ☐ Worrying about health because of the food allergies
- ☐ Worrying about eating a food even though everything indicates it is safe
- ☐ Worrying about being near foods because of the food allergy
- ☐ Feeling anxious about living with food allergy
- ☐ Feeling anxious or worried about an allergic reaction happening and/or treating it
- ☐ Not doing what I or my child wants to do because of food allergy
- ☐ Others are giving me trouble because of my food allergy
- ☐ Food allergy is affecting relationships
- ☐ Not wanting to undertake a doctor supervised oral food challenge test because of fear or worry

Emotional Concerns and Anxiety

What emotional concerns occur because of food allergies?

The most common emotion is anxiety. But people with food allergies and their families may experience fear, sadness, depression, and many other negative emotions.

When should anxiety be considered a concern for people with food allergies?

The first step is to consider the degree of anxiety and its consequences. Food-allergic reactions are serious, so it is normal and healthy to have some anxiety. In fact, it may be protective by increasing vigilance. For example, if the anxiety motivates a person to check ingredient labels and ask appropriate questions in restaurants, that degree of anxiety is healthy.

Signs of unhealthy degrees of anxiety may come out in various ways:

- Concerns that prevent you from eating in restaurants or at social functions
- Loss of sleep caused by thinking about your food allergy
- Rechecking foods you already checked and found safe
- Experiencing physical signs of anxiety and panic (sweating, shaking, heavy breathing, and so on) associated with meals and concerns about your food allergy, or seeing new negative behaviors in children
- Being in a heightened anxious state for more than a month after an allergic reaction

How should I address anxiety related to my food allergy?

Talk about the concern with your doctor. Anxiety disorders and phobias not related to food allergies can still affect food allergy management. It is helpful to diagnose this type of mental health problem because it can be treated and has no direct relationship to the food allergy. Whether or not the anxiety is related to food allergy, many approaches are available to help.

These include relaxation techniques, positive self-talk, distraction, and many others. If the anxiety is solely related to your food allergy, learning more about it, with emphasis on what is and what is not worth worrying about, may be helpful. For example, the unfounded worry that being near a food could cause a severe reaction may lead to unnecessary anxiety. Talk openly about your fears. When your anxiety is related to having experienced an allergic reaction, remember to focus on the positive aspects—that the reaction was recognized and treated, and that you learned from it. Sometimes additional tests, such as a food challenge or a touch test with a food, may allay concerns.

What is a "touch test" for food allergy?

I base the touch test on two studies I performed. In one study, I asked 30 children with severe peanut allergy to sniff peanut butter for 10 minutes, and I touched them with a pea-sized amount of peanut butter for 1 minute (see Simonte et al. in chapter 11). None of the children had a reaction to smelling the peanut butter (one had an anxiety response when smelling fake peanut butter, used as a placebo), and none had more than a minor itch or redness at the spot the peanut butter touched. Afterward, many of the children and families felt less worried about being around the food.

After the first study, we wondered how much doing a touch test could help people. We approached children ages 9–17 who expressed worries about being near or touching their allergen and were willing to be in a study that could include touching it (see Weinberger et al. in chapter 11). The child was randomly assigned to hearing about the study I mentioned above or doing that plus touching their allergen. It turned out that both approaches were equally effective in reducing their worries.

Can anxiety cause food allergy?

Anxiety itself does not cause the body to have a food allergy, but it can result in symptoms that mimic a food allergy. One way this can occur is through hyperventilation.

How does anxiety/hyperventilation mimic a food allergy reaction?

When people become fearful and anxious, they may not notice that they are breathing deeply and rapidly. Doing so alters the chemicals in the bloodstream, which can result in light-headedness, muscle cramps, tingling, numb fingers, and feeling as though it is hard to breathe. It can be difficult to know whether the symptoms are from hyperventilation or an allergic reaction when fear of a food exposure is part of the reason for the anxiety. I think that explaining this situation to people who have been having such symptoms often improves the problem through awareness. Anxiety counseling may be needed as well.

Can anxiety cause a person to appear to have a food-allergic reaction?

Absolutely. This is a reason why doctor-supervised feeding tests are sometimes designed to include placebo food, which does not contain the allergen being tested but looks, tastes, and smells like the real thing. This allows the testing to proceed with less bias. It can be difficult for a doctor or a person with a food allergy to know whether symptoms are from anxiety or represent a true reaction. Anxiety symptoms can include changes in skin color, trouble breathing, throat tightness, sweating, vomiting, and loss of consciousness. Some people get spasms of their vocal cords, causing wheezing sounds that mimic asthma. This problem goes by the name "vocal cord dysfunction." Such symptoms clearly overlap the symptoms of an allergic reaction.

The reason for anxiety is clear. Your body knows to fear the food that can cause a reaction. If someone held a gun to your head, you might shake, sweat, turn pale, have trouble catching your breath, and even pass out—clearly not from a gun allergy but out of fear and anxiety. This is a normal protective neurologic and hormonal reaction, but it can complicate food allergy diagnosis and treatment. If you or your doctor suspect anxiety reactions, this problem should be openly discussed and evaluated, and consulting a mental health professional should be considered.

Is there a link between food allergy and mental health problems?

There is no clear link between mental health disorders and food allergies. Some controversial reports link food allergies with depression, but more studies are needed.

Can food-allergic reactions cause increased anxiety? A posttraumatic stress disorder?

Yes. An allergic reaction can be a scary event that might cause increased anxiety for a time. This anxiety should naturally wane in days or weeks. If it does not, talk to your doctor. Sometimes a traumatic life event will lead to a more severe form of anxiety, a posttraumatic stress disorder.

Can food-allergic reactions result in fear of eating?

Yes. Sometimes people with food allergies begin to distrust the safety of various foods and may excessively limit their diet. Although this is a protective response, it is an example of an overreaction. Talk to your doctor about this if it should occur. Counseling is beneficial.

How should I address resistance to eating caused by anxiety in a child with a food allergy?

For a child, it should be helpful to emphasize that responsible adults are checking to make sure the foods are as safe as possible. Depending on the degree of concern and resistance in eating, it may be necessary to gradually reexpand the diet over weeks. Provide positive reinforcement. For a child, this may be a sticker chart, with a sticker for each small gain and rewards every so often for progress. Rewards should be given for even the smallest successes, and no one should dwell on times when progress is not made.

How should I address resistance to eating caused by anxiety in an adult with a food allergy?

For an adult, excessive dietary restriction may require a multidisciplinary approach, with counselors, allergists, and trusted friends ensuring that the diet is appropriately and safely expanded.

How can I handle sadness and depression related to food allergy?

It is normal to feel sad, helpless, or angry because of food allergies. It is not "fair" to have dietary restrictions and the constant concerns about allergic reactions. Also normal are feelings of guilt that arise among family members, who may feel as though they somehow caused the allergy. Some feel lucky not to have a food allergy, and then feel guilty for even thinking that. All of these feelings, if periodic and not interruptive of daily activity and social interactions, are normal. Talk about these feelings with friends, relatives, clergy, and professionals as needed. If the feelings are constant, overwhelming, or interruptive, however, you should seek professional assistance.

How should I address my general well-being as it relates to food allergy?

Although it is normal and expected that having food allergies, or having a family member with them, will result in concerns about general well-being, these feelings should not interfere with daily activities. Remember that people with food allergies can live full and happy lives while taking the necessary precautions to stay safe. This is the aspect that should be emphasized.

Is there a way to prevent anxiety, fear, and depression related to food allergies?

Not entirely, but there are healthy approaches that should reduce the risk of an overreaction to having a food allergy.

- Focus on the individual's positive traits. People are not defined by their food allergy. They are smart, creative, warm, friendly, artistic, athletic, compassionate, altruistic, and so on.
- Focus on allergy management successes. Emphasize the successfully obtained restaurant meal and the persistence in ensuring that activities are not curtailed by having food allergies.
- Address concerns early. If anxieties and fears are resulting in unnecessary alterations in lifestyle, address the problem quickly before poor habits set in.
- Avoid anxiety-provoking discussions around young children. Do not discuss dying from food allergies, turning blue, throat closing, or other scary terms. It is less troubling to use phrases like "could make you sick."

• Talk to your doctor about what you should and should not be concerned about. It is anxiety-provoking to be fearful of trace exposures that cannot be seen. Do you or your child need to be concerned about ingesting trace amounts? Do you or your child need to be concerned about touching or being near the allergens? Usually the answer to these questions is "no," and knowing this could allay anxiety.

When is it time to get professional mental health services to address problems caused by dealing with a food allergy?

In studies, more than 70% of people living with food allergies said they would benefit from mental health counseling (see Annunziato et al. in chapter 11). This high number reflects how difficult managing food allergies can be. Numerous studies have shown a significant change in quality of life. If you or your family are experiencing frequent and disruptive emotional concerns, discuss these concerns with your doctor and consider professional mental health services.

What do mental health professionals offer?

A proper mental health evaluation is important, and only a qualified mental health professional can provide an accurate diagnosis. You might attribute depression or anxiety to food allergy, but these can be independent illnesses or have different triggers (such as school phobia or generalized anxiety). Behaviors such as food avoidance may not be solely attributable to food allergy and may have components of anorexia or obsessive-compulsive disorder. The correct diagnosis is crucial to make sure the appropriate treatment is applied.

Mental health professionals can also provide counseling. A mental health professional might use cognitive behavioral therapy (CBT), a well-validated and frequently used psychotherapy that focuses on thoughts, feelings, and collaboration in an effort to reduce distress. CBT may combine food allergy education with self-monitoring (what is associated with feelings of distress and what coping skills help), coping skills training (relaxation techniques, distraction, problem-solving, positive self-talk), and social problem-solving skills (assertiveness training and recognizing problematic situations).

How would I recognize emotional concerns or anxiety in a young child?

A young child might have changes in behavior after an allergic reaction or another life event. The changes could be alterations in sleep patterns, increased aggression, defiance, expressions of sadness, reduced activities with family and friends, expressions of worry, and changes in eating. Discussion with your physician and referral to a mental health professional are options. Various techniques for counseling and therapy, including play therapy, are available (see www.a4pt.org).

Can food allergy cause mental illnesses like depression or schizophrenia?

No. Some people believe that foods cause various mental health problems through "allergy" or other effects. But there are no proven direct links. You should discuss such concerns with a physician or mental health professional, because altering the diet rather than addressing the problem through proper treatment can result in delaying effective treatment.

Interpersonal Relationships and Bullying

How do I address family relationships affected by food allergies?

It is not uncommon for management of food allergies to result in frustration among family members. Siblings may feel limitations caused by the diet restrictions. Relatives might not show the support that was hoped for in providing a safe environment. Sometimes relatives respond with disbelief about the allergy or feel that it should be addressed with fewer or more restrictions. Making sure everyone involved is fully educated about the allergy is helpful, especially to address questions about managing the allergy. The activities of siblings and other family members do not usually need to be restricted, but if this becomes necessary, it is fair to provide special occasions for them so that all the attention is not constantly focused on the allergy.

How should I address spousal relations that are affected by our child's food allergy?

Marital stress associated with managing a child's food allergies is common. Different parenting styles, varying levels of concern, or divergent preferences for managing the allergy can all put a strain on the relationship. If possible, both parents should attend office visits with the allergist to ask questions and determine approaches to care that are agreeable and safe. Talk about the disagreements without involving your child, and then favor a unified approach once the disagreements are aired.

How common is bullying of children with food allergies compared with those who don't have them?

One study showed that 50% of children with food allergies in grades 6 through 10 had experienced bullying, teasing, or harassment, compared with 17% without food allergies (see Lieberman et al. in chapter 11). The bullying was generally along the lines of taunting ("Ha, ha, I'm eating this, and you can't have any!"), provoking fear ("You drank from the water fountain after I rubbed peanut butter on it!"), or committing physical abuse (such as throwing peanuts or tainting a meal with allergen). Bullying has most often been attributed to peers, but adults and others may also be the perpetrators.

What are the negative consequences of bullying for a child with food allergies?

Being bullied does not make a person "stronger." Depression, low self-esteem, health issues, poor grades, and suicidal ideations are potential results of this victimization. For children with food allergies, the impact of bullying may be increased by the risks of a reaction when physical threats are involved.

Why is bullying more common for children with food allergies?

One possibility is that other children, or adults, are curious about the allergy and want to test boundaries.

How should bullying of children with food allergies be addressed?

Studies show that a child may not inform parents about food-related bullying, so parents need to raise the issue and discuss it with their child. In fact, one 2013 study showed that when parents were informed of the bullying, the child had less anxiety and better quality of life (see Shemesh et al. in chapter 11). When parents informed the school, bullying was more likely to end and the child's quality of life to improve.

Many schools have programs to address bullying or can invoke state laws on the matter. Table 7.2 shows advice based on articles written by Mati Sicherer, EdD, a school counselor with expertise in bullying.

Table 7.2. What to Do and Not to Do about Food Allergy–Related Bullying, Teasing, and Harassment

---

Recognize signs of bullying, including torn clothing or damaged books; unexplained injuries; school avoidance; physical complaints (headaches or stomachaches); consistent nightmares; declining grades or loss of interest in schoolwork; change in demeanor, with sadness or outbursts; and social isolation.

Be responsive and listen to your child. Stay calm. Reassure your child that you will help with this problem.

Do not confront the bully yourself. Parental intervention in bullying situations tends to exacerbate the problem. School personnel should have primary responsibility for managing the bully.

Do not encourage retaliation. Teaching your child to tease or fight back typically makes the situation worse. The bully is unlikely to be stopped by your child's response. Bullying is based on an inequity of power, so recurrent conflict allows the bully to display strength over your child. Encourage reduced contact with the bully.

Teach your child the difference between "telling" and "tattling." Tattling is done to get someone in trouble, while telling is done to get help. Encourage your child to promptly tell an adult about bullying.

Although the weight of responsibility should not be placed on your child, be proactive and teach assertive social skills. Role-play and practice ways to deal with the bully. Teaching your child how to say "Leave me alone" in a confident manner may be all it takes to stop a bully.

Inform and involve teachers, the principal, and other school staff. Do not assume that they know about the bullying. Many times, victims do not want to tell for fear of retaliation.

Set up a buddy system. Encourage your child to stay in a group of trusted friends in high-risk areas, such as in the lunchroom, during recess, and on the way home from school.

Encourage educational programs about food allergy and about bullying. Teachers, counselors, and school nurses may be able to provide lessons to increase food allergy awareness and reduce bullying.

Talk to your child's principal or school counselor about policies and plans regarding bullying. A typical approach is to initially observe the situation for a brief time and then take action. Serious consequences for the bully should be a part of the plan. Simple things such as moving the bully away from your child in class, not placing the bully in your child's class the following year, and staggering leaving times for the two children can be effective.

Nutrition

What nutritional concerns arise for an individual living with food allergies?

Depending on the number of foods avoided, concerns include whether there are sufficient calories, protein, carbohydrates, vitamins, minerals, and micronutrients (trace elements) in the diet.

Do food allergies cause weight gain or obesity?

No. There is a notion in the popular press that allergy, such as allergy to wheat, causes weight gain. Although avoiding wheat products such as cakes, cookies, and pasta might result in weight loss, this is not a sign of a true allergy.

Can food allergies cause weight loss or poor weight gain?

Yes, with three possible explanations: if there is inadequate energy (calorie) intake, increased energy needs that are not being met, or poor absorption of ingested calories.

Why would food allergies cause inadequate calorie intake?

Several reasons. There could be inadequate replacement of alternative foods during avoidance diets. Some illnesses may result in poor appetite and lower intake (for example, eosinophilic esophagitis). Sometimes anxiety about eating results in food avoidance or refusal or limited dietary intake.

Why would food allergies cause increased energy needs?

If there are severe skin rashes or inflammation of the gut, the body may need extra calories to make constant repairs.

Why would food allergy result in poor absorption of calories?

If allergens are causing inflammation in the gut, there can be reduced efficiency of the gut in absorbing needed nutrients.

Can food allergies cause poor growth in children?

Yes. Usually there is poor weight gain ahead of any reduction in height. There should be room for "catch-up" when the problem is recognized and addressed.

Are nutritional requirements different for people with food allergies?

No, but if there is ongoing severe eczema (atopic dermatitis), the child may require extra calories to continuously repair the skin damage. If gut allergies are causing poor nutrient absorption, additional nutrients may be needed until the digestive system heals.

What type of nutritional monitoring is recommended for persons on a food allergy elimination diet?

For children, their height and weight should be monitored on standard growth curves.

What nutrients are needed in the diet?

A healthy diet includes a proper amount of protein, fat, carbohydrates, vitamins, minerals, and trace elements. Caloric intake, the amount of energy from the diet, is an important consideration for proper growth. Calories are derived from the intake of protein, fat, and carbohydrates. In addition to energy, specific nutrients (vitamins, minerals) in the diet are needed to ensure proper body functions and to prevent illness.

Why are proteins needed, and how does food allergy affect protein intake?

Proteins are a source of the building blocks of life, amino acids. Good-quality proteins that include specific, much-needed "essential" amino acids are typically obtained from meats or complementary foods, such as the classic rice and beans, for individuals who are vegetarian or allergic.

What fats are needed in the diet, and how does food allergy affect fat intake?

Fats are a major source of calories, and essential fatty acids (linoleic and linolenic) are necessary for proper brain development in infants. These types of essential fatty acids are found in fish, which is often excluded from the diet of an individual with food allergy. These fatty acids are also available in vegetable oils, such as canola, corn, soy, safflower, and olive. The diet should consist of a blend of saturated fats, which are usually of animal origin, and monounsaturated and polyunsaturated fats, which are components of vegetable oils.

What carbohydrates are needed in the diet, and how might food allergy affect carbohydrate intake?
Carbohydrates, or complex sugars, are a major source of calories needed for growth, generally accounting for nearly half of the caloric intake. Vegetables, fruits, and grains contain carbohydrates. Wheat products are a common source of carbohydrates, but this food is a common food allergy. Substitutions for carbohydrates could therefore include corn, oats, potatoes, quinoa, and rice.

What additional dietary nutrients are needed in the diet?
Vitamins, minerals, and trace elements are necessary for various functions in the body, such as blood clotting, bone development, teeth development, proper nerve and muscle function, and many others. Examples of vitamins are vitamin A, which helps with growth and night vision, and vitamin D, which aids in the body's use of calcium. Examples of minerals are calcium, for bone development, and iron, which helps the blood carry oxygen through the body. Trace elements in the body include zinc, which is needed for healing and immune function.

What is the role of vitamin D in allergy?
Studies suggest that vitamin D deficiency may be a risk factor for allergy and that people with allergies may be more likely to be deficient in vitamin D. There is some evidence that vitamin D is needed to promote healthy immune responses. This does not mean that taking excessive supplemental vitamin D is warranted. Doing this could in fact be detrimental. The body naturally makes vitamin D when exposed to sunlight, and vitamin D is in many foods, but some of them are common allergens (eggs, fish, milk). Talk to your doctor about whether a blood test to check your or your child's vitamin D level is warranted.

What are alternative sources of nutrition for people avoiding allergens?
If you or your child are avoiding several foods, you should discuss your specific dietary needs with your doctor and possibly a registered dietitian. For infants, complete formulas are available to supplement any potential deficiency. Table 7.3 provides some examples of nutrients that may be affected by allergen elimination and suggests alternatives.

Keep in mind that the amount of nutrients in the alternative sources may vary greatly. For example, a calcium-fortified soy drink may or may not have "ounce-for-ounce" calcium levels similar to milk, and a calcium-fortified beverage likely has much more calcium per serving than a vegetable does. Be sure to discuss these substitutions with your doctor or dietitian.

How much carbohydrate, fat, protein, and other nutrients do I need for a healthy diet?

This varies with age. The US Department of Agriculture (USDA) maintains consumer-friendly documents regarding dietary recommendations at www.usda.gov. You can also check www.choosemyplate.gov.

Will my child get enough calcium on a milk-restricted diet?

Many beverages are fortified with calcium. Usually, children are not allergic to the various calcium-fortified fruit juices available, but calcium-fortified soy or rice drinks would also be a good choice and often have more calcium than the juices. It may be necessary to provide calcium as a supplement, for example, calcium carbonate tablets or gummies. Calcium and vitamin D needs change with age, so talk to your doctor or dietitian.

Does using soy drinks cause problems in boys?

There is some concern that phytoestrogens (plant-derived estrogens) as found in soy may have negative effects on men or boys. At this time, research studies fail to support this worry, and various professional organizations and government agencies have concluded that there is no need for concern.

Does food allergy cause picky eating in children?

No. Many young children have narrow food preferences with or without food allergies. But some children may develop food aversions (especially if they experienced an allergic reaction), and behavioral or feeding therapy may be needed.

When should consultation with a registered dietitian be undertaken for food allergy?

If there is any concern about a growth deficiency or when prolonged dietary avoidance is undertaken, a consultation is recommended. Since nutrient deficiency could occur despite normal growth, contact a dietitian if the diet is devoid of milk or other common foods, or if there is any suspicion that a restricted diet may be nutritionally inadequate.

Table 7.3. Nutrients Affected by Allergen Elimination, and Alternative Sources of Those Nutrients

Nutrient	Allergen	Alternative Sources
Calcium	Milk	Leafy green vegetables, beans, calcium-fortified drinks
Chromium	Peanut	Whole grains
Folate	Soy	Leafy green vegetables, beans
Iron	Wheat, soy	Meats, beans, dried fruits, iron-fortified grains
Magnesium	Soy, peanut	Fruits, vegetables, grains
Manganese	Peanut	Leafy green vegetables, whole grains
Niacin	Wheat, peanut	Meats, beans, enriched grains
Pantothenic acid	Milk, egg	Meats, fruits, vegetables, grains
Phosphorus	Milk, soy	Poultry meats, carbonated beverages
Riboflavin	Milk, egg, soy, wheat	Meats, leafy green vegetables, grains
Selenium	Egg	Meats, grains
Thiamin	Soy, wheat	Pork, beef, beans, grains
Vitamin A	Milk	Spinach, potatoes, squash, carrots
Vitamin B12	Milk, egg	Meats
Vitamin D	Milk	Fortified alternative "milks" and juices, margarine
Vitamin E	Peanut	Green leafy vegetables, vegetable oils, grains
Zinc	Soy	Meats, beans

What are the benefits of a nutritional evaluation for persons with food allergy?

There are several. The dietitian may have advice about products that are free of your or your child's allergens. The dietitian can also review a three-to-seven-day diet record to determine whether you or your child are obtaining the appropriate calories and balance of protein, carbohydrates, fats, vitamins, minerals, and trace elements needed for proper growth, health, and development. If there are potential deficiencies, substitutions could be suggested, such as using additional oils or seeking supplements in the form of multivitamins, iron, or calcium. It is vital to review any food allergies with your dietitian, so that appropriate substitute foods are selected.

Chapter Lessons

Jason has milk, peanut, and tree nut allergy. In the past year, his family explains, he has become more and more nervous about his allergies. He refuses to eat a packaged food until he has read the ingredient label several times. He worries that food residue from doorknobs, computer keyboards, and other surfaces may be on his hands, and he therefore washes his hands more than a dozen times a day. He worries that his mother may have forgotten about his allergy when she prepares his meals and sometimes refuses to eat unless she remakes the dish while he watches. His family has explained to him that they are very careful about making his food and that he should not have to worry about these "invisible" amounts of allergen, but he does not seem to trust them.

When I spoke with Jason and his family, it became clear that he worries about things more than necessary. However, encouraging him to trust his family and not worry was not going to be enough. There was also a family history of obsessive-compulsive disorder. Jason's actions suggested that he may also have this disorder and that his food allergy was simply a focus of his attention. Jason was referred to a psychiatrist who prescribed medications that helped Jason manage his food allergy with less stress.

Jane is a 16-year-old who has been avoiding milk, peanut, tree nuts because of her food allergies since around age 2. Over the past year, she has been complaining of increasing symptoms of gastrointestinal discomfort or itchy mouth from more and more foods. She has limited her diet and refused to have anything other than a few specific fruits, vegetables, and rice, and only in small amounts. She has lost weight and has become quite thin, worrying her family. Jane does not think she is "too thin," and she refuses to eat more because of her food allergies.

Upon evaluation by her pediatrician, allergist, and a gastroenterologist, no additional allergies were identified, and no gut issues were noted. Her body image and refusal to eat alerted her physicians to a diagnosis of anorexia nervosa. Treatment of this condition resulted in her improved health and weight gain.

Both Jason and Jane were attributing their behaviors to food allergy, but further evaluation determined other reasons. Successful interventions for both ensued. These case examples highlight the importance of getting additional help and not always assuming food allergies are a cause of the problems experienced by those with food allergy.

CHAPTER 8

The Natural Course and Resolution of Food Allergies

This chapter describes what we know about whether a food allergy is likely to resolve, as well as how food allergies occur in the first place. It also looks at the natural course of food allergies, including why some food allergies are more likely than other food allergies to go away over time.

General Questions about Food Allergy Resolution

Can food allergies resolve?

Yes.

Which food allergies are most likely to resolve?

Childhood allergies to egg, milk, soy, and wheat typically resolve.

Which food allergies are generally long-lived?

Allergies to peanuts, tree nuts, fish, and shellfish are typically persistent. Table 8.1 shows the natural course of common childhood food allergies.

Why is a food allergy outgrown?

The immune system is supposed to recognize, but generally ignore, the proteins in our foods. When a food allergy resolves, perhaps the immune system has altered the way it was recognizing the food. This might be because the immune system's cells eventually "forget" about attacking the protein. Another possibility is that the immune system has some chances to see the food protein again but does so in a healthier way. Perhaps during a time of earlier exposure, the immune system was irritable and set to

Table 8.1. Approximate Rates of Allergy Resolution in Childhood

Food/Food Group	Percentage Chance the Allergy Will Resolve (Be "Outgrown") during Childhood
Egg	85
Milk	85
Peanut	20
Seafood (fish and shellfish)	10
Soy	85
Tree nuts	10
Wheat	85

attack the new food, but later it is behaving appropriately and learns to ignore the food. Yet another possibility has to do with how the food is digested. An infant's gut may be more prone to let food proteins pass into the bloodstream. If the immune system is attacking undigested proteins but ignores digested ones, which often may be the case, then a child may outgrow their food allergy primarily because they are digesting the foods more effectively.

What predicts whether a food allergy will resolve?
There are no simple predictors, although having relatively lower food-specific IgE antibody levels in the blood is associated with a better chance of the allergy resolving, and early high levels are associated with less chance of resolution. Based on a series of studies, children under 2 years of age who have egg, milk, soy, or wheat IgE levels less than 2–5 kU_A/L typically lost their allergy before adolescence (reviewed in Savage et al.; see chapter 11). The relationships to IgE level are described more below. Infants with more severe eczema are less likely to resolve their food allergies early compared to those with mild or no rash.

Is there anything that can speed recovery from a food allergy?
The answer to this question is elusive. Some believe that strict avoidance speeds recovery, but this idea remains unproven. Children with milk or

egg allergy who can tolerate small amounts of these foods when they are extensively heated in baked goods, such as muffins, appear to have a better chance of outgrowing milk and egg allergies. Some children have anaphylaxis to these types of baked foods, so talk to your doctor.

The Course of Allergies to Specific Foods

What is the natural course of peanut allergy?
Peanut allergy is usually long-lived, although about 20% of children under age 2 with a peanut allergy will outgrow it by adolescence. Most of the resolution seems to occur by age 5 years.

What is the natural course of tree nut allergies?
Allergies to tree nuts are usually long-lived, but 5% to 10% of children diagnosed under age 2 will outgrow it by adolescence.

What is the natural course of milk and egg allergy?
Milk and egg allergies usually resolve in childhood. There is a very good chance (about 80%) that the allergy will resolve before age 5, although some studies suggest that the rate of outgrowing these allergies has slowed, with about half still allergic around age 9. Nonetheless, most children outgrow these allergies by adolescence. If the milk blood IgE test is more than 50 kU$_A$/L in the first years of life, the chance of resolution by adolescence is around 40%, and for egg with this level only about 15% resolved.

What is the natural course of soy allergy?
Soy allergy usually resolves in childhood. There is a very good chance (about 85%) that the allergy will resolve before age 5, although some recent studies suggest that the rate of outgrowing soy allergy has slowed, with about half still allergic around age 7. Nonetheless, most children outgrow this allergy by adolescence. Those with soy IgE levels above 50 kU$_A$/L in the first years of life had a resolution rate of 50% by adolescence.

What is the natural course of wheat allergy?
Wheat allergy usually resolves in childhood. There is a very good chance (about 85%) that the allergy will resolve before age 5, although some recent

studies suggest that the rate of outgrowing wheat allergy has slowed, with about half still allergic around age 6. Nonetheless, most children outgrow this allergy by adolescence. Those with wheat IgE levels higher than 50 kU_A/L in the first years of life had a resolution rate of 70% by adolescence.

What is the natural course of fruit and vegetable allergy?

Most fruit and vegetable allergies are associated with pollen allergies. They are usually mild, occur with the raw forms, and occur throughout adulthood. They can vary significantly depending on the pollen season, with more abundant pollen seasons triggering more symptoms when the fruit or vegetable is eaten. The natural course has not been studied well but likely varies significantly depending on pollen exposure.

What is the natural course of meat allergy?

This has not been studied, but it is possible to outgrow a meat allergy.

What is the natural course of fish and shellfish allergies?

These allergies are usually long-lived. The rate of resolution has not been studied well, but it is probably in the range of 5% to 10%.

The Course of Illnesses Caused by Food Allergies

Do food allergies that cause food protein–induced enterocolitis syndrome (FPIES) resolve?

Most often these resolve within a few years. Unfortunately, a small percentage of people continue to have this type of allergy for many, many years.

Do food allergies that cause eosinophilic esophagitis resolve?

Eosinophilic esophagitis appears to be a chronic disease that is usually not completely outgrown. The triggering foods could vary over time, so periodic reassessment is necessary.

Do food allergies that cause anaphylaxis resolve?

Yes, they can, according to the course of allergy associated with the individual food.

Does food-associated exercise-induced anaphylaxis resolve?

There are no good studies on this question. It may be related to the course of allergy to the causal food.

Does oral allergy syndrome resolve?

It varies in severity and triggers over time, but no studies detail how often the problem resolves completely.

Does atopic dermatitis (eczema) related to foods resolve?

Based on observations that food triggers of atopic dermatitis are uncommon among adults, it seems that this problem often resolves during childhood.

Evaluations for Resolution of Food Allergy

How does one know when a food allergy is outgrown?

The allergist performs tests to monitor for improvement. At some point, if there is significant improvement, a medically supervised feeding test could be performed to determine resolution. This test may also be offered if a circumstance indicates that the allergy might have resolved, for example, if an accidental ingestion did not result in any reaction.

What tests are performed to monitor for resolution of food allergy?

The two main tests are skin tests and blood tests that measure food-specific IgE antibodies. To monitor an allergy, the blood test is most convenient. Decreasing test results are often a good sign that the allergy is resolving, although, for young children, having results not increase is also a good sign. See chapter 3 for more details about allergy testing.

Why would a food allergy test increase or decrease?

We often see this despite no clear explanation. This question is addressed in detail in chapter 3.

How often should allergy testing be done to evaluate for resolution?

The factors that an allergist considers in retesting include the age of the child, the food involved, the time since the last reaction, and personal preferences and curiosity. Younger children might be tested with a higher frequency (perhaps every 6 to 12 months) than older persons because changes occur more rapidly. Some foods that are outgrown more readily, such as eggs, milk, soy, and wheat, might be tested more often than foods that tend to cause persistent allergies, such as fish, nuts, peanuts, and shellfish.

Recurrence of a Food Allergy and Development of New Food Allergies

Is it possible to redevelop a food allergy that is outgrown?

Yes, but this is unusual. A medically supervised feeding test is typically performed to confirm that a food allergy has resolved. When a medically supervised feeding of a food has a negative or tolerated result, people can generally eat that food for life. About 3% of the time, the test appears to have resulted in no symptoms, but problems arise in the days following. That is different from a situation in which a person with a negative feeding test has successfully consumed the food many times since. Once an individual is routinely eating the food, it is very unusual to have the food allergy recur.

Under what circumstances have food allergies redeveloped after resolution?

Since it is possible to develop a new food allergy at any time of life, an allergy that was outgrown could recur, although this is rare. One food to which recurrence of allergy has been well documented is peanut. Almost all recurrences of peanut allergy happened under similar circumstances. An individual successfully ingested peanuts during a feeding test but did not continue to incorporate peanuts in their diet afterward. The person then noticed symptoms many months or over a year later when trying to eat peanuts again.

If a food allergy resolved, how often does the food need to be eaten to prevent recurrence?

Although our experience with peanuts suggests that continuing to eat the food may be important, there are no established guidelines. I do not suggest creating a calendar for eating a food. Rather, when a new food is added to the diet after an allergy has resolved, incorporate it into the diet in a natural way. For peanuts, this might be a few times a month, and for foods like milk and eggs, it would be many times each week.

Why does a new food allergy occur in adults?

We do not know, but there are theories. The most common new allergy is to raw fruits and vegetables due to proteins in airborne allergens such as pollens. The food proteins are similar to the pollen proteins. Exposure to an airborne protein seems to trigger an allergy more often than exposure to an ingested protein, which may explain this situation. Another theory suggests that the adult's immune system might become vulnerable for a period after a viral infection or other illness. Still other theories suggest that changes in digestion may create a vulnerability. No one knows for certain why new allergies develop. See "Delving Deeper" at the end of this chapter for more on this topic.

Which food allergies develop in adulthood?

The foods that have most often been described as causing new allergies in adults are raw fruits and vegetables, as described above, as well as fish, peanut, shellfish, and tree nuts. Prevalence studies in the United States (Gupta et al. 2018 and 2019; see chapter 11) tracked the rates of children and adults with food allergies and asked the adults whether the allergy started in childhood and persisted, or was a newly occurring allergy during adulthood. The approximate rates of self-reported food allergies and the percentage of adults whose allergies started in adulthood are shown in table 8.2. It was surprising to see rather high percentages of adults reporting new-onset adult allergy to foods often thought of as childhood food allergies. More studies are needed to verify these reports.

Factors Affecting the Course of Food Allergies

Does the severity of an allergy affect resolution?

The answer to this is somewhat unclear because many children with severe reactions to foods such as egg, milk, soy, and wheat nonetheless outgrow these allergies. Compared with children who have consistently milder symptoms, however, persons experiencing more severe reactions, especially if they have strong positive tests, seem to experience a longer-lived allergy.

Table 8.2. Self-Reported Prevalence of Specific Allergies in Children and Adults and the Percentage of Adult-Onset Allergies

Food	Percentage of Children under 18 Years (Approximate)	Percentage of Adults 18 Years and Older (Approximate)	Percentage of Adults with Adult-Onset Allergies (Approximate)
Any	8	11	50
Egg	1	1	30
Fish	0.5	1	40
Milk	2	2	23
Peanut	2	2	18
Sesame	0.2	0.2	26
Shellfish	1	3	48
Soy	0.5	0.5	45
Tree nut	1	1	35
Wheat	0.5	1	53

Does being exposed to an allergen or having reactions affect the natural course?

Although it might be assumed that having exposures prolongs the allergy, this has not been proven. On the one hand, some studies show that recurrent exposures heighten allergic responses. On the other hand, studies aimed to treat food allergy have used exposure to attempt to reduce the allergic response. In a practical sense, a person with allergies must take all necessary precautions to avoid exposure, but our studies suggest that an accidental ingestion or purposeful exposure during food challenges does not significantly change the possibility of outgrowing allergy.

Delving Deeper

Why would an adult develop a new food allergy?

For adults, whose immune systems are supposed to be able to recognize but intelligently ignore food proteins, there appears to be a possibility of becoming allergic because of exposures that do not include eating. An example is baker's asthma, where occupational exposure to wheat protein results in wheat-induced asthma. Occupational exposures to other air-borne food proteins, such as milk and beans, have been reported. The most common example of new-onset food allergy is oral allergy syndrome, or pollen-associated food allergy syndrome, where allergy to pollen results in symptoms from eating raw fruits or vegetables that have similar proteins inside them. Another example where non-ingestion exposure triggers allergy is when an allergy to mammalian meat is triggered by tick bites, known as alpha-gal allergy (described in chapter 1).

Curiously, environmental allergens other than pollens share similar proteins to foods. Many tree nuts also have pollen-related proteins. Shellfish share proteins with dust mites and cockroaches, which are common environmental allergens. No one knows for certain, but this may be one reason why adults are more likely to develop these allergies, especially to foods that are eaten infrequently. The immune system may have time to develop an attack from the respiratory side, while the gut side of the immune system is not being exposed. Similarly, the skin may be a portal for allergy. The use of food proteins in cosmetics and skin care products may also provide an allergy-provoking exposure. A new onset of oat allergy has been attributed to using oatmeal baths. Milk, soy, and wheat allergies have also been traced to using skin care products, like soaps, with these ingredients.

Other possibilities to explain adult-onset food allergy have been theorized. Some cases of new-onset seafood allergy were described in adults using acid-blocker medications, the theory being that reduced digestion from using the medication might have allowed the allergen to trigger a response.

In summary, adult-onset food allergy is most likely attributable to having exposures that are not through eating the food, an explanation that has also been proposed for childhood-onset food allergy. It is likely that the individual's allergic predisposition/susceptibility plays a large role, but the lack of ingestion exposures and abundance of skin and airborne exposures to food proteins or related proteins likely drives the occurrence of adult-onset food allergy.

CHAPTER 9

Prevention of Food Allergies

Advice about preventing food allergy has changed radically in recent years, and it continues to evolve. In this chapter, I address questions about risk factors and how we may be able to prevent food and other allergic illnesses by reducing those risks.

General Questions about Risk Factors and Prevention Strategies

What are the risk factors for developing a food allergy?

Genetics (heredity) and environment are major factors.

How do genetics influence whether a person has a food allergy?

Genetics, or heredity, is how we pass along traits such as hair color or eye color. Heredity is also important for allergy. Although neither our genes nor our inherited genetic traits can be changed, knowing something about a person's genetic risk of allergy can help focus prevention on people who are at greater risk. Allergies are more likely to occur in a person whose relatives have allergic diseases, such as asthma, eczema, hay fever, or food allergies. The more types of allergies, and the more relatives with allergies, the more likely another family member will have them.

What is the risk of "inheriting" food allergies?

We do not know the exact risk of inheriting allergies to specific foods. My studies have found that siblings have a 7% risk of sharing a peanut allergy, which is about seven times higher than expected (Sicherer et al. 2000; see chapter 11). Another study that considered allergy to any food suggested that 14% of siblings share having food allergies (Gupta et al. 2016; see chapter 11). Still, many people who have allergies don't have any relatives who are also suffering.

If a person has nonfood allergies, are they at more risk of having a food allergy as well?

Yes. A personal history of any allergy increases an individual's risk for having additional allergies. The more allergic diseases, or the more severe the allergic disease, the more likely a food allergy will occur. Studies have found that if a child's allergic eczema is moderate or severe—meaning that half the body or more is affected with the persistent rash—the child has about a 35% risk of developing a food allergy (Eigenmann et al. 1998; see chapter 11). The risk of developing food allergy could be conceptualized based on family and personal history, as shown in figure 9.1. Personal history is a stronger risk factor than a family history. For example, a baby who has no eczema or signs of any allergic problems and has an older sibling with peanut allergy is at much lower risk than if that baby had eczema.

What are environmental exposures?

When we think about exposures and food allergy, the infant's diet usually comes to mind, and most of this chapter focuses on this topic. The world

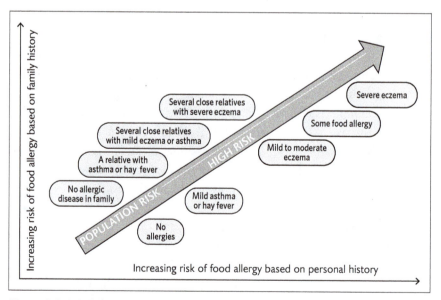

Figure 9.1. Family history and current personal history translate to risk of having or developing food allergies or having multiple food allergies.

of exposures is much more expansive than food choices, however, and can include environmental exposure to germs, chemicals, and other allergens. Later in this chapter, I address these factors. To complicate matters, environmental exposures can alter heredity (a process called epigenetics), leading to differences in risk for future generations.

How strong a role does the environment play in the risk of having a food allergy?

A very strong role. The apparent epidemic of food allergy that has occurred over the past 20 years has to be attributable primarily to the environment, not to genetics. In my study of identical twins who share the same genes, only 66% shared peanut allergy. If genes were the whole story, the rate of shared allergy would be 100%. Some type of environmental factor is responsible for the apparent rise in food allergy over the past several decades.

How would the environment affect having allergies?

The immune system, the part of the body that typically fights infection, is responsible for causing allergies, including those to food. The cells and chemicals that are designed to combat parasite or worm infections are also the ones that trigger allergies. Therefore a food allergy can be thought of as a misdirected response against foods from a part of the body that is ready to fight germs, especially parasites. One possibility to explain the rise in allergies is that changes in our lifestyle and environment have increased the risk of having them.

How would our environment cause the immune system to turn against us by attacking foods?

The "hygiene hypothesis"—also called the "old friends" theory or, more accurately, the effect of our communities of microbes that live in and on our bodies (the microbiome)—is one way to explain a rise in allergies and other diseases. Our lifestyle has left our immune systems without exposure to the "healthy" microbes that lived in balance with our immune system, leaving the immune system more prone to attack innocent proteins, resulting in allergy. We have avoided the "good" germs by living in cities rather than on farms, having smaller families and larger living spaces that reduce exposure to germs, living in clean houses and apartments, and using vaccinations, antibiotics, soaps, and other measures to stay healthy. Some studies suggest that birth by Caesarean section may increase the risk of developing allergies because the infant does not have exposure to the natural bacteria of the birth canal. Studies suggest a lower risk of allergy in children whose families do not use dishwashers—which extensively and thoroughly clean plates and utensils—and in parents who cleaned their children's pacifiers by sucking on them rather than washing them off, and thereby presumably passing more germs to the infant. Additionally, we have protected ourselves from parasite infections. The same parts of the immune system that fight parasites are active in creating allergies. Persons who are prone to allergy may have immune systems that would have been effective in fighting against parasites, but without parasites, the immune response may be prone to misdirected attacks on innocent proteins, like those in foods.

What role does dietary exposure to allergens play in the risk of having a food allergy?

The answer to this question is complex. On the one hand, an allergy cannot happen unless there is exposure to the proteins. You probably do not know anyone who is allergic to sluremi. The reason is that there is no such food as sluremi, and therefore no one can have an allergy to it. Acorn nuts would probably be a significant allergen, but they are too sour to eat, and so acorn allergy is not an issue (except, perhaps, for squirrels!). Allergy to rice is much more common in Japan than in the United States, which probably reflects Japan's higher rice consumption. Kiwi allergy was not described in the United States until these fruits were imported. On the other hand, the immune system is designed to recognize and ignore the food proteins that we eat, in a process called oral tolerance, so eating foods should normally not cause allergy.

Is it possible to prevent food allergies and allergic disease through diet?

Yes, but perhaps not in the way you might have guessed. Prevention of food allergies does not seem to be related simply to whether allergenic foods are included in the diet. Decades ago, there was a notion that delaying an infant's exposure to allergenic foods, such as egg, milk, and peanut, might reduce the risk of allergy, but newer studies refute this idea, and dietary recommendations have changed dramatically.

Why was there a notion that avoiding allergenic foods might prevent food allergy?

A number of studies showed that infants who were fed a milk-based formula had a higher risk of atopic dermatitis or milk allergy compared with those who were breastfed. A randomized study done more than three decades ago that had allergy-prone mothers delay giving their infants several allergens resulted in less observed milk allergy and eczema in the first year of life (see Zeiger et al. in chapter 11). These observations led to the idea that early exposure to whole proteins is a risk factor for allergy. Presumably, the young infant's immune or digestive system was ready for mother's milk, but not whole proteins. The observations from decades ago, and the notion that infants may not be ready for allergenic solids, resulted in the view that food allergies could be prevented by prolonged avoidance of common allergenic foods, such as eggs, fish, milk, and peanuts. Looking back at these studies, however, there are faults. The study that avoided giving infants allergenic foods early observed a delay in allergy onset but no long-term differences. And study results from decades ago may not apply to our modern lifestyle.

What are the new theories about the role of environment and diet with regard to food and other allergies?

New theories regarding risk and prevention of allergy and food allergies consider a complex interaction of genetics, environment, and immune responses. Here are just some examples:

- The "dual allergen exposure hypothesis" proposed by Gideon Lack, MD, identifies the skin as a route of exposure leading to food allergy. Infants with eczema (atopic dermatitis) are at increased risk for food allergy. Perhaps one reason for this is that exposure to foods on inflamed skin triggers allergic responses that can translate to allergic reactions when the food is eaten. Rather than following the notion that food allergy causes increased eczema, it may be that worse eczema is a risk for having food allergy because of the ease of becoming allergic through environmental exposure of the food on inflamed skin, especially if the food is not being eaten. Circumstantial evidence for this theory was found in one of our studies where peanut allergy was more likely in infants not eating peanut but living in homes with high peanut levels measured in the house dust; these infants were more likely to be affected by the household exposure to peanut if they had worse eczema (see Brough et al. in chapter 11). Additional evidence includes finding a higher risk of peanut allergy with specific genetic defects in the skin barrier and with using peanut-containing skin creams.

- Exposure to microbes is the explanation used in the "hygiene hypothesis" and the "old friends" theory. Countries with lower rates of allergy have more crowding, more animal exposure, lower rates of antibiotic use, lower rates of Caesarean sections, and so on. People living in those conditions are exposed to more microbes than are people living in less crowded conditions with less animal exposure, more antibiotic use, and higher rates of Caesarean sections.
- The role of dietary nutrients lies behind the "nutritional modulation hypothesis." Vitamin D, fatty acids, antioxidants, and folate have been the focus of this hypothesis, which offers primarily circumstantial and some conflicting evidence. These nutrients may affect the immune system. Regarding vitamin D, allergy rates appear to be higher in people who live farther from the equator (these people have less sun exposure, leading to less natural production of vitamin D from the skin, which requires sunlight). Omega-3 fatty acids have anti-inflammatory properties, and the proportion of these acids compared to nonprotective fatty acids has decreased in the modern diet, raising the question of their role in allergy. The nutrients in "diverse" diets and "healthy" diets may have advantages over unhealthy diets of prepared foods with unhealthy fats.
- There are other hypotheses, too: the obesity and diabetes epidemics, food additives and preservatives, vaccination (related to hygiene), chemical treatment of crops, genetically modified foods, climate change, and other factors have been considered as potentially contributing to the increase in food allergy. There are a host of theories regarding why we are seeing more allergy and food allergies specifically. Many aspects of the modern lifestyle have changed during a period where allergy and other diseases have increased. Although some reasonable considerations underlie the various theories, the theories are inconclusive because of conflicting evidence or missing evidence.

Many of the above hypotheses are explored further later in this chapter.

What strategies to prevent allergies have been studied?
Studies have addressed the following aspects of the mother's or infant's diet:

- The mother's diet during pregnancy
- Whether the infant is breastfed or formula fed
- The role of the mother's diet if breastfeeding

- The type of formula used if formula feeding
- The timing of introduction of solid foods
- The timing of introduction of specific common allergens, especially eggs, milk, peanut, tree nuts, and wheat

Additional studies have evaluated other dietary factors and active forms of prevention that do not involve the allergenic foods per se, such as probiotics (health-promoting bacteria), dietary nutrients, and other factors.

Pregnancy Diets

Can a mother's diet during pregnancy protect her infant from allergy?
A handful of studies have specifically addressed the impact of peanut ingestion during pregnancy. Several small studies of highly allergic young children showed a relationship between a mother's ingestion of peanuts during pregnancy and her child's peanut allergy. In contrast, several larger studies of children overall, not just those who were allergic, did not show a relationship.

Analysis of the multiple available studies of several foods concluded that a mother's dietary exclusion does not appear to prevent allergy in children and carries a risk of fetal malnutrition (see Netting et al. and de Silva et al. in chapter 11). The analyses include a study of more than 2,500 German children focused on the maternal diet in the last four weeks of pregnancy that related the diet to eczema and "food sensitization" at the child's second birthday. The study found no relationship between the mothers' dietary intake of eggs, milk, or nuts and the allergy outcomes. Interestingly, maternal intake of margarine increased, and intake of fish decreased, the children's risk of eczema. This finding may be related to having "good fats" in the fish and "bad fats" in the margarine, which affect immune responses. It is notable that fish, a worrisome allergen, was protective of allergies. A study of 1,277 mother-child pairs from the United States, who were not selected for any specific disease, found reduced rates of allergy in children whose mothers ate higher amounts of milk, peanut, and wheat in early pregnancy. Overall, there appears to be no strong evidence that a mother's restriction of allergens during pregnancy helps prevent allergy in her child, although there is some controversy.

What do experts recommend regarding a mother's diet during pregnancy for allergy prevention?

Numerous recent US expert panels (in 2008, 2010, 2013, 2017, 2019, and 2020) and international expert panels (in 2008, 2015, 2016, 2017, and 2020) that evaluated the available evidence reached similar conclusions, and do not recommend food allergen avoidance diets during pregnancy for the purpose of preventing food allergies.

If there is controversy about the benefit of avoiding peanuts during pregnancy, why do the experts not err on the side of saying to avoid it?

Expert panels have shied away from making recommendations when the available evidence is unclear. The scientific community simply does not know the best answer and would not want to give advice that may turn out to be wrong or harmful. Individual families, however, can always use the available information and their own experiences to make choices. Some families have excluded peanuts from their home because of family members with peanut allergies. Some families find it easier to exclude an allergen to reduce the risk of accidentally ingesting it. In this situation, a pregnant mother is already unlikely to ingest very much. For her, it may be sensible to follow a diet that is already in place. Statements from the expert panels are not specifically recommending that peanut be increased or excluded from the diet, so a pregnant mother should feel at liberty to manage her diet as she sees most reasonable.

Breastfeeding and Formulas

Does breastfeeding prevent food allergy?

There are many reasons to breastfeed, and exclusive breastfeeding is encouraged for the first four to six months of infancy, with some guidelines suggesting exclusivity to about six months. Studying the role of breastfeeding on food allergy is difficult because, first, studies cannot randomize infants to breastfeeding—that is, assign some infants to breast and some to bottle. A second reason is that the many factors that influence a mother's decision on how long to breastfeed and whether to breastfeed exclusively can bias conclusions about the relationship between breastfeeding and allergies. A 2019 clinical report from the American Academy of Pediatrics,

Table 9.1. Breastfeeding and Allergic Disease

Allergic Disease	Conclusion
Eczema in the first two years of life	Decreased risk from exclusive breastfeeding for the first three to four months
Wheezing in the first two years of life	Any duration of breastfeeding beyond three to four months is protective, irrespective of duration of exclusivity
Asthma even after age 5	Some evidence that longer duration of any breastfeeding, as opposed to less breastfeeding, is protective
Food allergy	No conclusions can be made about the role of any duration of breastfeeding in either preventing or delaying the onset of specific food allergies

which I coauthored, made several conclusions based upon the available evidence regarding breastfeeding and allergy outcomes. The report concluded that there are no short- or long-term advantages for exclusive breastfeeding beyond three to four months for prevention of allergic disease, and additional conclusions are summarized in table 9.1.

Can a mother's diet during breastfeeding prevent allergies?

Few studies address this question, and some are ongoing. It is known that a tiny amount of ingested protein can pass into breast milk. For some infants, that amount can induce allergic symptoms. But it is not clear whether this type of exposure, for most infants, is a potential means of causing an allergy or, perhaps, a natural way to teach the infant's immune system to accept various foods. If it is the latter, then a mother's diet may play a role in preventing allergy by including rather than excluding foods. Based on the few available studies, allergen avoidance during breastfeeding of an otherwise healthy infant does not appear to prevent allergic disease.

What do expert panels recommend regarding a mother's diet during lactation for allergy prevention?

The US and international expert panels recommended against mothers' avoidance of allergens during lactation as a means to prevent food allergies. I advise a diverse and healthy diet for the breastfeeding mother. If an infant is experiencing illness that could be attributed to the maternal diet during lactation, an evaluation for allergy is recommended, but this is different from a prevention strategy in an otherwise healthy infant.

What is the role of infant formulas in preventing food allergies?

Some infant formulas are derived from cow's milk or soybean. Typical formulas have whole proteins, similar to proteins in whole cow's milk or soy. Some infant formulas have predigested cow's milk proteins. This improves digestibility (partially hydrolyzed) or can make the formula safe for children with milk allergy (extensively hydrolyzed formula). There are also specialized formulas made from amino acids, the building blocks of proteins, and these are nonallergenic. No studies have found that infant formulas are superior to breastfeeding for prevention of allergy.

Although breast milk is the best choice, are any infant formulas useful in preventing allergy?

Although some early studies suggested that specific infant formulas, the hydrolyzed formulas, may prevent allergy, the weight of the evidence over decades suggests this is not the case. The 2019 American Academy of Pediatrics Clinical Report and the 2020 Consensus Statements from the United States and Canada, as well as multiple international guidelines, have concluded that these formulas do not prevent allergic disease, even in those at high risk.

What is the current approach to infant breastfeeding or formula feeding to prevent allergies?

In summary, experts recommend exclusive breastfeeding for the first four to six months of life, with some suggesting exclusivity to around six months.

Introducing Solid Foods

When should a baby eat solid foods?

The timing of introducing solid foods is partly related to the length of exclusive breastfeeding, as mentioned above. While exclusive breastfeeding is recommended by some authorities to 6 months, many add complementary foods from 4 to 6 months. Solids cannot be started until an infant is developmentally ready to swallow them, typically starting around 3 months. An infant should have good head control and be able to eat while upright. Of course, the consistency of the food matters. Infants under 6 months typically manage pureed foods, moving to semisolid/lumpy foods around 8 or 9 months and toward small soft-solid finger foods around 12 months. Nuts or thick nut butters are considered choking hazards. There is currently no convincing evidence that delaying solids, including potentially allergenic ones, for prolonged periods prevents food allergy, and doing so may actually increase the risk of developing an allergy.

What would be a possible exception to allowing an unrestricted diet for an infant who is prone to allergies?

If an infant is already showing signs of allergy, there may be additional potential allergens that could trigger reactions if offered. For example, an infant who already showed evidence of milk allergy or has experienced serious allergic rashes is at increased risk of having an egg or peanut allergy. In this situation, you should discuss additional allergen introductions with your doctor. For an infant who is otherwise well, there is a lack of evidence that waiting longer is protective.

Should allergenic foods be introduced "early"?

In the United States, parents traditionally introduce grains first, followed by vegetables and then fruits. This progression is not related to allergy. Many physicians recommend waiting several days between trying different foods because of concerns about allergy or intolerance, but this is also a traditional approach rather than one based on any specific studies and can potentially unnecessarily delay a varied diet, including allergens. Various cultures introduce different foods in different sequences. Foods that are more difficult for an infant to safely ingest, such as choking hazards like pieces of meat, nuts, and so forth, by default must be introduced later, when a baby is able to manage them without choking. But recent studies have suggested that at least for peanut, likely egg and possibly other foods, there can be a protective advantage to introducing these allergens early.

What evidence suggests that feeding peanut early may prevent peanut allergy?

Experts generally agree that based on one very good study there is compelling evidence that feeding high-risk infants peanut early may reduce their risk of peanut allergy. The study, performed through a single hospital in London, was called the LEAP (Learning Early About Peanut Allergy) study, and it evaluated infants 4 to 11 months of age who already had severe eczema and/or egg allergy (see Du Toit et al. in chapter 11). The study excluded infants with strong positive allergy skin tests, assuming they were already allergic to peanut. The remaining infants were randomly assigned to one of two groups: one group ate a large serving of peanut about three times per week from the time they enrolled in the study through to age 5 years, and the other group avoided peanut. The study found that the rate of peanut allergy was 17% in those who avoided peanut compared to 3% in those who ate peanut early. Among infants entering the study with negative allergy tests, there was an 86% reduction in peanut allergy, and for those with small positive allergy tests, there was a 70% reduction in peanut allergy. A later study had the infants avoid peanut for a year, and it appears that the benefit was sustained. The approach did not appear to interrupt breastfeeding or affect nutrition.

What questions remain from the study about feeding peanut early?

Unanswered questions include: How would the study performed in London translate to other countries? What amount and frequency of peanut are needed? What type of testing is best to identify those at risk at the time of first feeding, and what level of medical supervision is needed? What are the risks of trying this approach outside of a study? What if a baby started and then stopped for a while? Is that riskier than just waiting? Would this approach be applicable to infants who have less sign or no sign of allergy? How long is it necessary to include peanut in the diet?

What about feeding other allergenic foods early?

A study called the EAT study (Enquiring About Tolerance) attempted to introduce cow's milk protein, egg, peanut, sesame, wheat, and white fish into the diet of breastfed infants from 3 months of age (Perkin et al. 2016; see chapter 11). These foods were introduced in succession and for a specified length of time, starting with milk protein and ending with wheat, randomizing the order of the other foods in between. The study, performed in England, did not focus on high-risk infants, although the families, who volunteered for the study, tended to have more allergic problems than average. Participating families were randomized to this early introduction group compared to a group who had a standard introduction of solids after 6 months of age. The results of the study remain a bit difficult to interpret. Overall, the group with early introduction of these foods did not have a significant difference in rate of any food allergy at 1 to 3 years of age. It was difficult to follow the diet, however, and when looking only at infants who successfully ate the required amount of the food, there was a reduction in peanut and egg allergy in the early-eating group. Five studies from Australia, Germany, and Japan attempted to introduce egg in the forms of a pasteurized egg-white powder, or a special heated whole-egg powder (the Japanese study), into the diet early in infants starting around 4 to 6 months of age (reviewed in Perkin et al. 2020; see chapter 11). The qualifications to be included were different in each study, so they included infants with eczema, infants without any particular allergy risks, and infants with a family history of allergy but without eczema. Three studies could not show that this approach reduced egg allergy, and one of them suggested increased risk, but they did note that many of the infants were already allergic to egg when they started the study, suggesting that if the approach worked, it may be necessary to start earlier. The Japanese study showed that the approach was effective, but the investigators tested the infants with the same special heated whole-egg powder they used during the study, rather than regular cooked egg. When the information from the EAT study and these additional five studies were combined, the analysis favored introducing egg early. But doing so would possibly go against the recommendation to exclusively breastfeed for four to six months, with many experts advocating breastfeeding for around six months. Studies on milk have also provided conflicting results. One Japanese study of newborns at risk of allergy (see Urashima et al. in chapter 11) suggested that exposure to cow's milk in the first three days of life increased risks for milk allergy, while another Japanese study (see Sakihara et al. in chapter 11) suggested that early and consistent exposure to cow's milk formula from 1 to 3 months of age reduced the risk of milk allergy. Additional studies are ongoing and planned. Translating these various findings into recommendations is discussed in the next section.

Current Recommendations

How have the recommendations about allergy prevention through diet changed over time?

Recommendations have changed dramatically and are still evolving. In 2000, the American Academy of Pediatrics recommended that mothers with a family history of allergy consider avoiding peanuts during pregnancy and allergenic foods during lactation, then not introduce milk until age 1 year; egg until age 2; and peanuts, tree nuts, and fish until age 3. The experts explained that these recommendations were not based on specific evidence from studies, but that they seemed reasonable given the state of knowledge at the time. All these recommendations were overturned in 2008. The committee on toxicology in the United Kingdom recommended similar restrictions on peanuts around the same time but also withdrew those recommendations. Various other expert panels from Europe and other countries never dictated specific allergen avoidance for the mother or infant. This left a passive type of comment on prevention, concluding that delayed allergen introduction would not prevent allergy and that allergens could be introduced as early as 4 to 6 months, but not specifically recommending that they be introduced early.

In the past several years, expert panels from different groups worldwide have offered guidance on allergen introduction for the purposes of food allergy prevention, with some differences among recommendations. Some of the reasons for discrepancies in advice stem from the willingness of various expert panels to provide guidance when the evidence is suggestive but not certain. Some advice suggests allergy testing in specific situations where the infant might be at risk of already being allergic, while others do not. Those who advocate for allergy testing prior to feeding the food feel that when the risk is already high, the testing may identify infants at risk for a reaction. Those who advocate against testing worry that the tests might "over-call" the allergy, result in more delays in trying the food, be impractical and costly regarding access to health care, and argue that it would be exceptionally rare to have a serious allergic reaction while trialing new foods.

What are the current recommendations about the timing of peanut introduction?
Early in 2017, a report of an expert panel sponsored by the National Institute of Allergy and Infectious Diseases (NIAID) was released (see Togias et al. in chapter 11). The report contains three guidelines that serve as an addendum to a larger report from 2010. The recommendations are summarized as follows:

1. Infants at "high risk." Infants with severe eczema and/or egg allergy should have infant-safe forms of peanut-containing foods introduced as early as 4 to 6 months of age (after the infant demonstrates that he or she can handle solid foods). The expert panel recommends strongly considering an allergy evaluation with testing to peanut to determine whether introduction is possible and recommends medical supervision for introducing it. Although 4 to 6 months of age is the target, the approach still applies for infants who were not introduced to peanut and are older than 6 months.
2. Infants with mild to moderate eczema should have introduction of infant-safe peanut-containing foods around 6 months of age in accordance with family preferences and cultural practices after other solid foods are introduced to show readiness. An in-office evaluation is not recommended but may be considered.
3. Infants without eczema or food allergy should have age-appropriate peanut introduced freely together with other solids and in accordance with family preferences and cultural practices.

   The first recommendation regards high-risk infants who are most likely to become allergic to peanut and is based largely on the results of the LEAP study, while the second two recommendations are extrapolated on the basis of expert opinion, but they also are in accordance with the results of the EAT study described above.

What type of allergy evaluation might happen prior to starting peanut?
For the infants at high risk because of severe eczema or food allergy, allergy skin testing is preferred because such testing was the most predictive of allergy outcomes in the LEAP study. However, the recommendations allow for allergy blood testing to peanut because blood tests are more widely available to primary care doctors. Testing to multiple foods is strongly discouraged (see chapter 3). If a blood test is positive, referral to a specialist is

advised. Depending on the test results, it might be concluded that it is "too late," that peanut allergy is likely already present and peanut needs to be avoided; or it may be concluded that peanut allergy is so unlikely that it can be added at home; or it may be "in between," with a conclusion that peanut be introduced under medical supervision either at the infant's usual pace of eating or, if there is a higher risk for allergy, in a graded oral food challenge (see chapter 3). As noted above, some experts and some guidelines suggest against pretesting altogether.

What is the feeding regimen for peanut?

The recommended feeding regimen for peanut follows the one tried in the LEAP study for high-risk infants, specifically 6 or 7 grams of peanut protein over three or more feedings each week. The LEAP study had the children do this to age 5 years. Special instructions for home feeding are directed only to the infants at high risk who underwent allergy testing but who are still considered reasonable candidates for home introduction. Those instructions are paraphrased in box 9.1, but your physician should provide specific directions. Box 9.1 also includes options for infant-safe forms of peanut, since peanuts and peanut butter are choking hazards for infants.

What about early introduction of allergenic foods other than peanut?

In the United States, fruits, grains, and vegetables are traditionally the first solid foods. First foods must have a consistency that is manageable for infants, so choking hazards such as nuts are not typically given early. Although the American Academy of Pediatrics recommendations from 2019 indicated that there is no convincing evidence that delaying intro-ductions of allergenic foods (such as eggs, fish, milk, and nuts) prevents allergy, early introduction was not specifically advised, except for peanut per the NIAID guidelines described above. The jury is out on the efficacy of earlier introduction, except for the likely benefit of peanut and possible benefit of egg as described above. This has resulted in some evolution of recommendations worldwide as more evidence accumulates.

What are the current international guidelines for starting allergenic foods?

Table 9.2 summarizes selected international recommendations from 2017 through early 2021, abbreviated to highlight specific aspects. While there are many similarities in these guidelines and recommendations, it is no-table that different groups have come to slightly different conclusions and approaches. The similarities are more striking than the differences, however. The primary theme is not to treat common allergens (egg, milk, peanut, wheat, etc.) much differently than other foods, and to not specifi-cally delay introduction. Especially for children with some increased risk, including allergens in the diet around 6 months of age is sound advice. It should also be appreciated that advice to purposefully avoid allergens for prolonged periods as an approach to prevention is no longer recom-mended by any group. If you did not get around to trying peanut for your 11- or 12-month-old, or if you did not introduce all allergens by 9 months of age, that does not mean "all is lost."

What is the latest approach for starting allergenic foods in the United States and Canada?

The latest consensus approach in the United States as of 2021 (Fleischer et al. 2021; see chapter 11) is included in table 9.2. Grains, fruits, and veg-etables are usually the first solid foods. First foods must be a consistency that is manageable for infants, so choking hazards such as nuts are not typ-ically given early. Talk to your pediatrician about introducing solids. For-tified infant cereals are often among first solids, to meet requirements for iron and zinc. Allergens are not introduced until the infant has been able to tolerate several more typical first foods. Regarding allergens, the 2021 approach highlights introducing peanut and egg around 6 months, reflect-ing most of the available data, and not delaying other allergens based on a lack of data that show harm of introducing them early even though proof of effectiveness of early introduction has not been determined. The ap-proach describes the potential for allergy testing and medically supervised feeding, but it is not required. As described previously, early introduction is generally safe, and pretesting may create barriers to early ingestion. For high-risk infants, the guidance recognizes that some families may prefer, in discussion with their allergist, to perform pre-introduction testing, which can be individualized. In studies that I and others have performed, we found that some families are reluctant to introduce allergens early. This tells me it is important to discuss the options with your pediatrician and allergist. For an infant without severe eczema or any known food allergies, it is difficult to argue for pre-allergen introduction testing, even if there is a family history of allergy.

BOX 9.1. FEEDING INFANT-SAFE FORMS OF PEANUT FOR PREVENTION OF PEANUT ALLERGY IN A BABY AT "HIGH RISK"

Below are instructions for introducing peanut at home to infants who are considered to be at risk for an allergy based on severe rashes or food-allergic reactions but who have been approved by their doctor to begin introduction of peanut at home.

Preparation

1. Feed your infant only when he or she is healthy; do not do the feeding if there are any signs of illness.
2. Give the first peanut feeding at home.
3. Make sure at least one adult will be able to focus full attention on the infant.
4. Make sure that at least one adult will be able to spend at least two hours with the infant after the feeding, to watch for any signs of an allergic reaction.

Feeding

1. Prepare a full portion of one of the peanut-containing foods from the recipe options.
2. Offer a small part of the peanut serving on the tip of a spoon.
3. Wait about 10 minutes.
4. If there is no allergic reaction after this small taste, then slowly give the remainder of the peanut-containing food at the infant's normal pace of eating.

Symptoms of an Allergic Reaction (see chapters 1 and 4)

Symptoms may include a rash, hives, swelling, vomiting, difficulty breathing, wheezing, repetitive coughing, changes in skin color (pale or blue), and sudden tiredness, lethargy, or limpness.

IF YOU ARE CONCERNED ABOUT YOUR INFANT'S RESPONSE TO PEANUT, OBTAIN IMMEDIATE MEDICAL ATTENTION OR CALL 911.

Recipe Options

Each recipe contains approximately 2 grams of peanut protein. Note: teaspoons and tablespoons are US measures (5 milliliters and 15 milliliters for a level teaspoon and tablespoon, respectively). Any of these meals should be fed about three times each week.

Option 1. Bamba

Bamba was the product used in the LEAP study and therefore has proven efficacy and safety. Other peanut puff products with similar peanut protein content may be substituted. New products are likely to be developed over time.

Infants should be fed 21 pieces of Bamba, which provide approximately 2 grams of peanut protein.

(a) For infants younger than 7 months of age, soften the Bamba with 4 to 6 teaspoons of water.

(b) For older infants who can manage dissolvable textures, unmodified Bamba may be fed. If dissolvable textures are not yet part of the infant's diet, softened Bamba should be provided.

Option 2. Thinned Smooth Peanut Butter

(a) Measure 2 teaspoons of peanut butter (9 to 10 grams of peanut butter; ~2 grams of peanut protein), and slowly add 2 to 3 teaspoons of hot water.

(b) Stir until the peanut butter is dissolved, thinned, and well blended.

(c) Let cool.

(d) Increase the amount of water if necessary (or add infant cereal that the infant already eats) to achieve a consistency that is comfortable for the infant.

Option 3. Smooth Peanut Butter Puree

(a) Measure 2 teaspoons of peanut butter (9 to 10 grams of peanut butter; ~2 grams of peanut protein).

(b) Add 2 to 3 tablespoons of pureed tolerated fruit or vegetables to the peanut butter. Increase or reduce volume of puree to achieve desired consistency.

Option 4. Peanut Flour and Peanut Butter Powder

Peanut flour and peanut butter powder are two distinct products that may be interchanged because they have similar peanut protein content per 10 grams of product.

(a) Measure 2 teaspoons of peanut flour or peanut butter powder (4 grams of peanut flour or 4 grams of peanut butter powder; ~2 grams of peanut protein).

(b) Add about 2 tablespoons (6 to 7 teaspoons) of pureed tolerated fruit or vegetables to flour or powder. You may increase or reduce volume of puree to achieve desired consistency.

Source: Adapted from Togias et al. (see chapter 11).

Table 9.2. Selected International Recommendations from 2017 to Early 2021 (Abbreviated)

Country and Year	Organization	Foods	Advice	Allergy Testing Advised before Offering Food
Australia, 2017	Australasian Society of Clinical Immunology and Allergy	Cooked egg, peanut, nut, wheat, fish	At around 6 months, but not before 4 months, start a variety of solids starting with iron-rich foods while continuing breastfeeding. All infants get allergens in first year of life. Infants with severe eczema or egg allergy should be given peanut before 12 months (good evidence). Cooked egg before 8 months may reduce egg allergy (moderate evidence).	No, unless the child already has a food allergy. If so, discuss peanut testing with the doctor.
Japan, 2017	Committee for Japanese Pediatric Guidelines for Food Allergy	Peanut	Wean at 5–6 months. Peanut at 4–10 months.	No
Great Britain, 2018	British Society for Allergy and Clinical Immunology / Food Allergy Specialist Group of British Dietetic Association	Egg, peanut, tree nuts, dairy, fish, shellfish wheat	Breastfeed exclusive for around 6 months. Infants with eczema or existing food allergy: solids including cooked egg and peanut (egg first) from 4 months, followed by other allergens. Other infants: solids around 6 months but not before 4 months, including allergens eaten as part of the family's normal diet.	No

Table 9.2 (cont.)

Country and Year	Organization	Foods	Advice	Allergy Testing Advised before Offering Food
Europe, 2019	European Food Safety Authority Panel on Nutrition, Novel Food and Food Allergens	Egg (cooked), cereals, fish, peanut	No evidence that early introduction increases risk, can introduce along with other complementary foods. Peanut introduced in the first year of life.	No
United States, 2019	American Academy of Pediatrics	Egg, peanut, fish, others	No evidence to delay beyond 4–6 months to reduce risk. Follow 2017 NIAID Guidelines for peanut. Data less clear for timing of egg introduction.	In selected cases for peanut (severe eczema and or egg allergy)
United States and Canada, 2021	Consensus of US and Canadian allergy societies	Peanut, egg, others	Introduce (peanut, cooked egg) to all infants regardless of risk starting around 6 months, not before 4 months. Once introduced, regular ingestion should be maintained. Do not deliberately delay other allergens.	Screening (pre-allergy testing) not required, remains an option

What are practical ways to introduce allergens early?

Peanuts and peanut butter are choking hazards for infants, and box 9.1 provides advice to create infant-safe forms. As mentioned previously, the old adage of introducing a new food every five to seven days is impractical. Unless there are signs of problems, a new food, including allergens, might be introduced every day or two, and once known to be tolerated, it can be continued and combined with new foods. When it comes to the amount of allergen that can induce "prevention," we have limited data. The EAT study suggested that relatively large amounts of egg or peanut were needed to have a prevention effect, but extensive studies are lacking. Similarly, the necessary frequency of ingestion is not known. It is likely that the amount and frequency differ by risk of allergy. Numerous companies have developed products with various allergens in infant-safe forms such as liquids, powders, and finger foods. These provide a quick and convenient format to introduce allergens that are not choking hazards. A 2020 review article by my colleague Marion Groetch, MS, RDN, from our Jaffe Food Allergy Institute and her dietitian and allergist colleagues, discussed the relative benefits and unknowns of these products (see Schroer et al. in chapter 11). Highlights of that review are shown in table 9.3. The commercialized products add a high level of convenience, but with a cost. At this time, products other than peanut (in amounts recommended by NIAID guidelines) are not proven to prevent allergy, and the US Food and Drug Administration does not support claims that they can be helpful in allergy prevention.

Nondietary Aspects of Prevention

Aside from allergen-related diet restrictions, how else might one prevent allergies?

Most of the attention regarding allergy prevention has focused on allergenic foods in the diet. Studies are underway to try to find other ways to prevent allergies, and these focus on identifying risk factors that could be modified, such as the following targets:

• *Skin barrier.* Studies suggest there is a relationship between eczema and a poor skin barrier to food allergy, as described earlier in this chapter. This observation would support the idea that aggressive treatment of eczema early on, or prevention of eczema, may reduce the risk of food allergy.

Table 9.3. Comparison of Convenient Infant Allergen Products versus Conventional Food

	Examples	Cost	Ingredients
Products marketed for infant allergen introduction	Single ingredient or mixed ingredient powders, liquid pouches, crackers, "puffs," etc.	Expensive (for peanut, about $9 to $30 per month; for egg, about $8 to $50 per month)	Caution about multiple ingredients if there is a preexisting allergy to one of them; generally low in calories and additional nutritional value; some products contain very small doses of allergen compared to doses recommended in guidelines; degree of heating/processing may affect food in ways that differ from conventional foods
Conventional foods	Peanut butter, peanut powders, Bamba, scrambled egg, milk, fish, nut butters, etc.	Inexpensive (for peanut, about 50¢ per month; for egg, about $1 to $3 per month)	Can source the specific allergen; often has broader nutrient quality; can adjust dosage; cooked as the natural foods

Several small, early studies of early skin treatment showed promise, but two large studies published in 2020 did not show effectiveness in preventing eczema.

- *Obesity.* Obesity has been associated with an increased risk for allergies, positive tests to food allergens, and asthma, although the relationship is unclear. Perhaps children with food allergies eat more calorically enriched foods, or, more likely, since obesity is associated with a state of increased inflammation, this inflammation might bias the immune system toward allergy. There are currently no studies proving this relationship.
- *Vitamin D deficiency.* As discussed earlier in this chapter, vitamin D is beneficial for healthy immune responses. There is evidence from several studies that vitamin D deficiency is associated with increased food allergy or positive tests to foods. Not all of the studies support this association, and

there is also some evidence that the effect of vitamin D deficiency differs depending upon hereditary aspects. A 2020 review from the European Academy of Allergy and Clinical Immunology found no support for the hypothesis that vitamin D supplementation reduces the risk of developing food allergy. The conclusion does not alter the suggestion to treat a known vitamin D deficiency, and additional studies are ongoing.

- *Poor intake of healthy dietary fats.* As mentioned previously, a diet with immune system–promoting fats from fish rather than fats from margarine may be beneficial. A balanced, healthy diet and lifestyle are likely important aspects of prevention. A 2020 review by the European Academy of Allergy and Clinical Immunology concluded that fish oil supplements during pregnancy, when breastfeeding, or in infancy may not reduce the risk of food allergy. They noted, however, on the basis of one study that when taken during pregnancy and during breastfeeding, it may reduce food allergy slightly in young children at increased risk.

- *Folate and other nutrients.* There have been concerns that folate supplementation in pregnancy to reduce the risk of spinal cord problems in newborns may increase allergy risks, but expert review of the data failed to show a relationship. Single uncontrolled reports suggest that antioxidants in the diet may be protective of food allergy, but expert review concluded that the studies are insufficient to draw conclusions because such studies suffer from biases.

- *Food choice and diet diversity.* There are insufficient studies to comment on the role of food additives, preservatives, or genetically modified foods as a risk factor for food allergy or on the potential benefits of organic food for "prevention" of allergy, although these products have been discussed as factors. Overall, evidence is lacking. Except for convenience and expense, arguments other than allergy risks might suggest food choice based on increasing "healthy foods." Studies find that infants who ate diets rich in fruits, vegetables, and home-prepared foods have less food allergy. Mediterranean diets (rich in fish, fruits, vegetables, legumes, nuts, and cereals) have also been associated with less allergic disease. The available information suggests a benefit to a diverse diet (Venter et al. 2020; see chapter 11).

- *Hygiene.* The increasing rate of allergy may be associated with improved hygiene, leading to misfiring of the immune system. Although use of antibiotics may be blamed, strong direct evidence is lacking. To address the possibility that a lack of exposure to germs is at fault, research has turned to providing exposure to health-promoting bacteria—probiotics as well as dietary nutrients that "feed" good bacteria, termed prebiotics.

- *Genetic/immune propensity to allergy.* We have much more to learn regarding why some infants and not others develop food and other allergies. As mentioned earlier, a genetic predisposition to make an allergic response is part of the propensity to allergy. Future approaches may look to treatments such as "biologics," medications that block allergic pathways.

Do probiotics and prebiotics prevent allergies?

Probiotics are live bacteria thought to have health-promoting effects. Prebiotics are indigestible food substances that help our bodies maintain these health-promoting bacteria. Increasingly, studies are evaluating the use of prebiotics and probiotics for prevention of allergic disease. There are many different types of probiotic bacteria, and their effects may vary. Some studies have suggested that early use of probiotics may reduce the risk of allergic eczema. Concerns regarding probiotics include the possibility of having an infection from them or having a reaction to milk contamination, because many of them are grown in milk. Based on limitations of the available studies and conflicting results, most expert panels have not recommended probiotics or prebiotics for food allergy prevention. A 2020 review by the European Academy of Allergy and Clinical Immunology considered eight studies on this topic and concluded that these have little to no effect on food allergy prevention, but the evidence is uncertain. As studies have identified specific communities of "good" bacteria associated with a reduced risk of allergic disease, studies are testing the idea of giving these mixtures to infants early on to determine whether they can prevent allergies.

If my child has allergies, can I do something to prevent new ones?

Unfortunately, children who develop a food allergy or any allergic disease are at risk for developing others. The "allergic march" refers to the observation that young children with allergic eczema or food allergies are at increased risk to "march on" to develop allergic asthma and hay fever. Although research is underway, we currently do not have any proven means to reduce the risk aside from those mentioned previously.

How can an adult with food allergies avoid getting new ones?

We do not have any sure ways to avoid new food allergies. Studies suggest that treatment of the pollen allergy with immunotherapy (allergy shots) may help some people to reduce symptoms from the related fruits or vegetables (oral allergy syndrome). Immunotherapy is usually suggested when hay fever is not responding well to medications such as antihistamines, medicated nose sprays, and eye drops. For persons undergoing immunotherapy, an added benefit may be reduced symptoms from the foods that are related to pollens. Not all studies support this observation, but it may be an extra benefit of having pollen immunotherapy for some people. Presumably, this treatment would prevent additional related fruits or vegetables from becoming problematic, but this is unproven.

Chapter Lessons

Toni is a 5-month-old whose parents brought her to see me because she has severe eczema. Her parents were interested in preventing peanut allergy, a problem her 3-year-old brother has been living with. Based on the current recommendations, and the favorable potential to avoid peanut allergy through early introduction, I discussed our options. If feeding peanut to Toni could be accomplished, they would need to commit to giving it to her at least three times per week. We discussed that they would need to ensure her brother did not accidentally eat peanut, which would now be in the home. We discussed that the introduction of peanut to Toni is not a guarantee that she will avoid future allergy, just a means to reduce the risk. Also, they had to make a long-term commitment to follow through with these feedings consistently for years. They were interested in doing this.

We discussed whether to pretest, and given their experience with her brother, they preferred this approach rather than trying peanut at home on their own. I performed a skin test to peanut, and it was positive, with a bump size of 4 millimeters. I explained to the family that there is a potential for current peanut allergy. We decided to have her introduce peanut under my direct supervision. There was a risk of reaction, but typically such reactions, if they occur, are not severe. Toni had not started any solids yet, and I needed them to introduce some so that I knew she would be able to take the infant-safe form of peanut without choking. They spent a week feeding her a rice cereal and jarred fruits and returned to the office. The oral food challenge went well, and I gave the family instructions to continue giving 6 to 7 grams of peanut over three or more feedings per week using infant-safe forms of peanut-containing foods. I will follow her until she is 5 years old, and then decide whether they can stop the high frequency of feeding peanut.

CHAPTER 10

The Future Is Now
Treatments for Food Allergy

One treatment for peanut allergy approved by the US Food and Drug Administration (FDA) is now in use, and additional treatments are likely soon to be available. Food allergy research is likely to find new ways to treat and hopefully even cure food allergy in the future. This chapter explores these topics: what is new in treating food allergy, and what promising avenues of research are being explored.

General Questions about Food Allergy Research

What are the goals of research in food allergy?

There are many research goals, such as determining how many people are affected by food allergy, risk factors, prevention strategies, better means of diagnosis, and of course better treatments. Additional areas include how to better educate people about managing their food allergies and improving quality of life. This chapter focuses on research for better treatments and cures.

What types of research currently address treatment of food allergies?

There are two broad categories of research: studies done in the laboratory and studies done in people. There are two types of approaches to treatments as well. One type is directed toward a particular food, such as peanuts or eggs, and would work only for that specific food, and another approach is to find a therapy to work for any food allergy.

What are clinical trials?

Clinical trials are ones performed in people to determine whether a therapy is safe and effective.

What are the prospects for future therapies to treat food allergies?
The future looks bright. Many ideas are being evaluated in the laboratory, and numerous clinical trials are evaluating various treatment options.

Who funds research on food allergies?
Research studies are funded in many ways. Your tax dollars may pay for studies through grants from the National Institutes of Health. Donations directly to researchers or through organizations that raise money for research are another source of funds. Pharmaceutical companies also fund research studies. Still, a major hindrance to progress is the lack of funding to allow the many good ideas for laboratory and clinical studies to progress.

Who regulates or supervises research on food allergies?
Research studies are regulated or supervised in various ways. If a study involves animals, institutional committees monitor the animals' welfare. When studies involve people, review boards address the safety and the scientific quality of the study. Clinical studies often require an ongoing review board not associated with the study to evaluate safety and progress. Additionally, if the study involves a drug or a medical device, there is an additional review by the FDA. In some cases, additional committees that address safety and scientific value will review a study, depending on the treatment being performed and the source of funding. The review process includes various experts and laypersons who ensure that the study is done safely, for good reasons, and that it is sensitive to participants who may be especially vulnerable, such as children.

How are research advances in food allergies reported?
Researchers generally publish their findings in research journals. The reports undergo evaluation by experts before being published. Preliminary reports are often communicated at scientific meetings. The general public usually hears about research advances through the media. It can be confusing to know whether the research result is significant or immediately applicable. Talk to your allergist if you believe you might benefit from some new finding.

How do scientists interpret their food allergy research results?
Carefully! It can be difficult to come to conclusions if a study suffers from limitations, and most studies are not perfect. The best type of studies

randomize people to a type of treatment and have a "fake" treatment (a placebo) so that those on a treatment and the people evaluating them do not know who is on the therapy being tested.

When does a research result cause a change in food allergy management?

Most research studies add small pieces to a larger puzzle. As evidence mounts, it is easier for people to be confident that the results are true and that a treatment or approach may be worthwhile. Often, the research on a particular topic from several different studies is analyzed together to ensure that the overall results from numerous studies are truly identifying a benefit (an approach called a meta-analysis). The available information is also evaluated by experts, often government agencies, and others to recommend changes in practice. Sometimes, the evidence remains unclear, and experts must choose whether to recommend a specific approach. Additionally, your doctor might consider the available evidence and your specific circumstances in making treatment decisions. For a new approach or treatment to be widely available and accepted, as well as covered by insurance, the approach typically must go through extensive phases of study to assess the risks and benefits as well as the effectiveness.

What types of basic science research are underway for food allergies?

Many laboratory studies evaluate the basic mechanisms underlying food allergies, trying to understand how and why the immune system "attacks" foods as well as various means that might interrupt or reverse that process.

What types of clinical studies are underway to treat food allergies?

The two main types are those that are designed to treat an allergy to any food and those that are focused on the treatment of a specific food (for example, just milk or just peanut).

What are examples of food allergy treatments that are not specific to particular foods?

Treatments that block immune responses.

What are examples of food allergy treatments that are specific to particular foods?

Examples include exposing a person to the food to which they are allergic, or a modified form of that food, in gradually increasing amounts (immunotherapy).

How do I keep abreast of what studies are underway and what progress has been made in food allergy therapy?
This is a fast-moving area, and although this chapter gives updates and insights on current treatments, you will need to talk to your doctor about what is currently available. There are many additional resources (see chapter 11) that provide information on research progress.

Which food allergy treatment under study is most likely to work in the long run?
We do not know which treatment will win out as safest and most effective. It is promising that numerous therapies are being tested, and the first ever FDA-approved therapy for a food allergy was approved for use starting in 2020. A particular therapy may be beneficial for some people but not others, and treatments may need to be individualized.

Approaches to Treat Any Type of Food Allergy

What is anti-IgE therapy for food allergies?
Most severe food allergies with a rapid onset of symptoms are triggered by the body producing IgE. In anti-IgE therapy, a protein is injected that essentially ties up and inactivates the IgE. The theory behind the treatment is that inactivating the body's IgE will reduce the risk of allergic reactions to any food. The drug is omalizumab, which goes by the brand name Xolair. This treatment has been in use for chronic allergic asthma and chronic hives that have not responded well to other therapies.

What have studies shown for using anti-IgE therapy for food allergies?
The studies have so far shown that most people on this type of therapy can generally ingest more of the food than when they are not treated. Not all people experience an improvement, however, and the degree of improvement varies.

What are potential advantages of anti-IgE therapy for food allergies?
The fact that the treatment can address any food allergy is a great advantage. Being able to increase the threshold at which a person reacts could reduce the danger of small exposures for sensitive people.

What are potential problems with anti-IgE therapy for food allergies?
There are several. Some people make so much IgE that the treatment cannot overcome it and cannot be used at all. The treatment itself sometimes causes an allergic reaction. Even for those who had some benefit, the therapy does not seem to completely block allergic reactions.

What is the status of anti-IgE therapy for food allergy?
Studies are underway to better characterize the effectiveness and safety of this approach, and we are hoping for FDA approval. In addition, the approach is increasingly being used in combination with treatments directed to specific foods (see below). Additional anti-IgE therapies using slightly different drugs that may have additional advantages in safety and effectiveness are under study as well.

What are Chinese herbal remedies for food allergy?
Traditional Chinese medicine has been used for centuries to treat many conditions, but food allergy historically was not one of them. Preliminary studies in people with food allergies have shown safety, but more needs to be done to understand if there is effectiveness.

What are probiotics, prebiotics, and synbiotics?
Probiotics are live microorganisms that, when administered in adequate amounts, confer a health benefit. Prebiotics are nutrients that help the healthy bacteria grow and survive, and "synbiotics" refers to the use of both at the same time.

How might probiotics, prebiotics, and synbiotics treat food allergies?
By providing health-promoting bacteria, researchers hope the immune system will become better balanced and less likely to attack innocent proteins.

What is the status of research on probiotics, prebiotics, and synbiotics for food allergy?

Regarding treatment, the results have been unclear. Most studies so far have not shown an effect, but research is ongoing, including combining probiotics with other specific therapies (such as oral immunotherapy), with the hope of improving their effectiveness. The correct choice of bacterial communities to promote treatment may need fine-tuning, and such studies are underway. Fecal transplant is another potential treatment that is being studied. See chapter 9 for the role of microorganic and nutritional supplements in the prevention of food allergy.

What are anti-cytokines, monoclonal antibodies, or "biologics"?

Anti-IgE, described above, is one example of a medication created or engineered from natural sources such as people, animals, or bacteria, also called a biopharmaceutical. Many of these drugs, typically given by injection, are proteins called antibodies that can attach to and activate or inactivate various components of the immune system. These drugs may attack chemicals or proteins used by the immune system (cytokines), or components of cells involved in immune responses. Other biologics may generally enhance "good" rather than allergic immune responses. There are many such products being tested for treatment of allergic diseases, but few are currently targeted to food allergy. But some of these new drugs, which may show promise in treating asthma, eczema, and other allergic problems, may eventually be tested in food allergy as well, whether for prevention or for treatment. These are extremely promising therapies because they could target multiple foods with the simplicity of a monthly injection. Table 10.1 reviews some of these agents, some of which are already approved for asthma or eczema, and many are being looked at for a variety of allergic diseases.

Approaches to Treat Allergies to Specific Foods (Immunotherapies)

Why are there allergy shots for pollen and environmental allergies but not food allergies?

"Allergy shots," or immunotherapy using injections, are effective for pollen allergies and allergies to stinging insects. They seem to work by reeducating the immune system not to "attack" the injected proteins by exposing a person to small and increasing amounts over weeks and months. In the 1980s, studies were begun using peanuts for injections. The treatment made it possible for the participants to eat larger amounts of peanuts, but the side effects of the treatment were too strong; people had allergic reactions, sometimes severe ones, to the allergy shots, and the strategy was abandoned.

Table 10.1. Selected Biologic Agents with Promise to Treat Food Allergy

Type/Name	What It Does and Why It Is Being Studied	What's Known So Far
Anti-IgE (omalizumab [Xolair] and others under study, including ligelizumab)	Inactivates IgE (used for asthma and chronic hives) Should increase threshold of allergy to any food/multiple foods	Raises threshold variably May allow for faster specific allergen immunotherapy and with fewer side effects
Block IL-4 receptor alpha (dupilumab [Dupixent])	Blocks various allergic pathways (already used for asthma and atopic dermatitis) May improve threshold or facilitate immunotherapy	Studies underway for using alone or in combination with immunotherapy
Block IL-33 (etokimab)	Interrupts an immune chemical (cytokine) that activates many allergy-related pathways	Improved threshold of peanut allergy in one small study
BTK inhibitor (ibrutinib)	A cancer drug that may also block responses of allergy cells	Preliminary study on a small number of people showed temporary blunting of food allergy tests
Other anti-cytokines (anti-IL-5, anti-TSLP, anti-IL-13)	Like etokimab above, many immune chemicals are involved in allergy pathways, and blocking them may have a role in tempering food allergy	Under study for asthma and atopic dermatitis ahead of food allergy

What are the different strategies for immunotherapy or allergy shots for food allergies?

The primary approach is to expose the immune system to the food proteins without triggering allergic reactions. Different strategies to do this include altering the proteins to make them less potent for triggering a reaction and more capable of promoting protective responses, or giving the proteins in a manner other than through an injection—for example, by mouth or on the skin—so that severe reactions to the treatment are less likely. There are studies looking at boiled (rather than roasted) peanut as a possibly safer form for immunotherapy. There are studies looking at injecting tiny amounts of peanut into lymph nodes, hoping to trigger strong protective immune responses without as many side effects. Proteins are also being engineered without parts that are more potent, chopped into smaller pieces that are less allergenic, or treated in ways that alter their structure to enhance effectiveness and improve safety. The treatment can also include proteins or other compounds that promote nonallergic reactions and target the treatment to the immune system in a way that promotes treatment (these are called adjuvants).

What is the status of research on vaccines for food allergies?

This is an extremely active area. The goal is to improve safety over simply exposing a person to a food allergen (which can cause anaphylaxis), while also promoting effectiveness. Here, we distinguish vaccination strategies from what will be described later as immunotherapy using unaltered food. These are not like childhood vaccines that prevent illness—they are directed to treat current illness. Peanut is the target of most of the studies at this time, but the strategies can be adjusted to any food allergy once safety and effectiveness are obtained. While we typically think of vaccines as being injected, strategies are also considering routes such as nasal or oral administration. Table 10.2 summarizes vaccine approaches. There are many approaches not reflected in the table, including strategies where food allergens are attached to molecules that promote healthy immune responses, strategies where altered allergens (to make them less likely to induce reactions) are combined with various additional molecules to promote anti-allergy responses, strategies where engineered antibodies against the allergen are injected, and many others.

Table 10.2. Selected Vaccine Strategies to Treat Food Allergy

Vaccination Strategy	Why It Should Work	Status
ARA-LAMP-Vax, a DNA vaccine	The vaccine does not contain peanut proteins Immune cells take up the vaccine and produce peanut proteins, priming the immune system to accept peanut	In safety studies in people
EMP-123, an engineered, less allergenic peanut protein encapsulated in a bacterium	The peanut protein should be less allergenic, so it should have fewer side effects Given as a rectal vaccine, the bacteria carrier may promote safety and a helpful immune response	In safety studies, some participants still had allergic reactions Further studies on hold
HAL-MPE1, a peanut protein that is partly digested and in a vaccine with alum adjuvant	The peanut protein should be less potent and the vaccine components should help induce healthy immune responses	Safety studies completed Efficacy trials planned
Glucopyranosyl lipid A (GLA) combined with peanut sublingual immu-notherapy	GLA should promote healthy and more robust immune responses to the low-dose sublingual peanut protein	Study was terminated
Peptide-based vaccine (PVX-108)	Specific segments of peanut proteins that stimulate pro-tective immune responses are injected into the skin Should have increased safety because only small segments of peanut are used	Safety studies
Nanoparticle-based therapeutics, with allergen and adjuvants	Nanoparticles are like tiny capsules that can hold various molecules As a delivery system, it may allow targeted combined therapies	No human studies yet

What are oral and sublingual immunotherapies?
Oral immunotherapy (OIT) or sublingual immunotherapy (SLIT) involves gradually giving the allergic food by mouth or as an extract under the tongue, respectively. Typically, a dose is given to an allergic person under medical supervision, and then the dose is continued daily at home until a slightly higher dose is given under medical supervision. The gradual increases in dosing are usually stopped when a targeted daily dose is reached. The target dose for OIT is larger than the target dose for SLIT. This strategy has been described in the literature for many decades. But *do not try this at home! Reactions can occur!*

Does oral immunotherapy or sublingual immunotherapy permanently cure a food allergy, or only change how much food can be eaten while the person is taking treatment?
The goal of the treatment is to allow a person to ingest more of the allergen than they could without treatment, a result called "desensitization." It remains under investigation whether this approach to treatment can be more like a "cure," meaning that the allergy is gone even when the daily dosing is ceased, a result called permanent "tolerance," "remission," or "sustained unresponsiveness." It is often impractical for a person who has undergone OIT with success (desensitization) to avoid ingesting the allergen for long periods.

Most studies, unable to test for a cure by having the individual stop eating the food for long periods such as a year, instead have participants stop therapy for one to three months and then assess whether they are still protected. If they remain protected, they are considered to have "sustained unresponsiveness." Whether success in ingesting the foods after a period of no treatment should be considered a cure is a point of controversy.

So far, OIT studies suggest that most people lose protection (desensitization) with suspension of dosing. This can occur even after a few days early in treatment, but loss of desensitization occurs more gradually if treatment stops after longer periods on therapy. In a peanut OIT study conducted at Stanford (see Chinthrajah et al. in chapter 11), after two years, 85% of participants were desensitized after ingesting 4,000 milligrams daily; with discontinuation of therapy for three months, only 35% could still ingest this amount, and a year later, only 13% could. Most studies have not compared the results of longer periods (years) of treatment, which may induce more permanent changes. Sublingual immunotherapy, which is not as robust as oral, has not shown a strong promise to induce a prolonged protection off therapy.

What is the status of treatment using sublingual immunotherapy for food allergies?

The studies thus far have been promising in that allergic reactions to the therapy are generally mild and uncommon, and persons on the treatment experience an increased threshold compared to those treated with placebo. The improvement has generally not been strong enough for most people to eat regular servings of the food, however, and many people experience rather small or sometimes no improvements. This is still a promising therapy that remains under study, including the possibility of adding additional co-treatments to improve the effectiveness, since the safety profile is already very good. Studies are also underway using variations on this approach, such as toothpaste or dissolving films (like some breath mints) that contain peanut protein.

What is the status of treatment using oral immunotherapy for food allergies?

In 2020, the FDA approved the first treatment for a food allergy, a peanut OIT (peanut allergen powder) called Palforzia. This is the only currently available FDA-approved OIT. It is approved to start from ages 4 years through 17 years. Once the child starts the treatment, they may continue it past age 17. This may seem like a narrow approval given that it is only for peanut and only for a specific age range. This reflects the studies that resulted in gaining approval. Multiple studies are ongoing to understand more about OIT, however. In addition, clinical practices have been taking up this approach not only for peanut but also for other foods.

What benefit can be expected from treatment with Palforzia or peanut OIT?

The primary benefit is to increase the threshold of reactions. Different studies have set different goals, studied a variety of dosing regiments, and aimed for a variety of final daily "maintenance" amounts to be eaten. A 2019 review looked at 12 peanut OIT clinical trials with 1,041 participants and concluded that those treated, compared to placebo, had about a 12-fold increased chance to tolerate more peanut (of various amounts) at the end of therapy (see Chu et al. in chapter 11). In one 2018 study specifically of Palforzia, in children 4 through 17 years of age, where the final daily does is 300 milligrams (equivalent to about one peanut kernel—there are usually two peanut kernels in each peanut shell), about 67% entering the study were able to ingest 600 milligrams of peanut with no more than mild symptoms (compared to 4% in the placebo group), and about half were able to eat 1,000 milligrams (compared to only 2.4% treated with placebo). Children eligible the study had to react to 100 milligrams or less during a supervised oral food challenge (see Vickery et al. in chapter 11).

What side effects can be expected from treatment with Palforzia or peanut OIT?

The 2019 review of 12 trials mentioned above concluded that that those on OIT had a little over threefold increased chance of anaphylaxis and just over twice the risk being treated with epinephrine compared to those not treated. Palforzia allergic reactions can occur at any phase of treatment (see below) but are most common during the time that dosing is being gradually increased. During that time, about 67% have stomach pain, 37% vomiting, 40% throat irritation, 32% cough, 33% itch, and 9% anaphylactic reactions (less than 1% had severe anaphylaxis). The major warnings provided for the treatment regard anaphylaxis, gut symptoms that can be chronic or recurrent, and development of eosinophilic esophagitis (EoE). In Palforzia studies, 2.7% were referred for suspicion of EoE, and ultimately 12 of 709 on Palforzia were biopsied and had EoE compared to none on placebo. There is not a clear risk assessment for EoE because a major reason for discontinuing treatment is gut symptoms, and referral for biopsy is not usually done. Stopping the therapy is typically associated with resolution. In studies of Palforzia, 22% on treatment stopped the therapy, with side effects being the reason to stop for 9%, mostly from gut symptoms. Side effects tend to decrease with time, but anaphylaxis can occur even on the final daily dose, even after the dose was tolerated many times.

What is the process of being treated with Palforzia?

The process starts with a discussion about goals, risks, and benefits. In addition, practical considerations about costs, time involvement, motivation, and practicality should be undertaken. We will discuss this more below. The actual process follows four stages.

1. *Preparation.* A thorough discussion with your allergist, your child, and family about how the therapy may be a good fit (or not). The approach trades the goal of raising a threshold of reaction to peanut against potentially having more allergic reactions than avoidance of peanut. Understanding this concept and being ready and willing to use epinephrine for an allergic reaction to the treatment is therefore vital. The FDA and the company making Palforzia have set up a Risk Evaluation and Mitigation Strategy (REMS) system (see www.palforziarems.com) that requires allergist prescribers, health care settings, pharmacies, and, importantly, patients to enroll. For patients, this includes understanding the risks and process, especially the importance of having self-injectable epinephrine readily available, and knowing how and when to use it for signs and symptoms of anaphylaxis. Additionally, patients must acknowledge that they will undergo monitoring with doses and avoid peanut other than the treatment doses.

2. *Initial dose escalation.* This is undertaken under direct medical supervision in a setting prepared to monitor for and treat allergic reactions. The health care professional administers five increasing doses from about 1/600 of a peanut to about 1/50 of a peanut, given every 20–30 minutes. The peanut powders come in capsules, which are opened and the contents mixed with small amounts of refrigerated or room-temperature soft foods such as applesauce, pudding, or yogurt. This process, which includes at least an hour of observation at the end, should take about 4–6 hours depending upon any symptoms. The process is abandoned if significant symptoms (those that warrant the use of epinephrine, for example) should occur. To go to the next stage (up-dosing), the 3-milligram dose (the fourth dose) has to be tolerated. The next stage ideally starts the next day, because if it is delayed more than four days, the initial dose escalation day must be repeated.

3. *Up-dosing.* This stage starts with a 3-milligram dose (about 1/100 of a peanut). There are eleven dose levels: 3, 6, 12, 20, 40, 80, 120, 160, 200, 240, and finally 300 milligrams. The start of each dose level involves the dose being given in a medical setting under direct supervision and monitoring. If tolerated, it is given at home daily for at least two weeks until the visit for the next dose level. At home, the dose is mixed as described above from specific capsules (there are four types of capsules used at home with different colors of capsule and writing on them, with guidance about what to use each day, and depending on the dose

level, one to six capsules may need to be opened each day). The dose is taken around the same time of day with a meal. The in-person visits will include at least one hour of monitoring after the dose, but it could take much longer if there are symptoms or concerns. If no dose modifications are needed (see below) and the schedule is followed with minimal interruption, the next stage may be reached in about 20 weeks.

4. *Maintenance*. The final dose, 300 milligrams, comes in a sachet rather than a capsule. The initial dose is given as an up-dose, but after that, if all goes well, this dose is given indefinitely.

Dose modifications (or discontinuation of treatment) may be needed during up-dosing or maintenance if reactions occur or if too many dosing days are missed. This could include going back to lower doses or staying on a current dose for a longer period. Sometimes daily doses are withheld for a few days on purpose if there are special circumstance, such as an illness (see below).

What are the daily "rules" for taking Palforzia?

Be sure to review expectations and instructions with your doctor. Some of the daily aspects are summarized here.

- Be sure you are comfortable with monitoring at home and knowing when and how to use medications to treat symptoms, including the use of epinephrine.
- Store the doses in the refrigerator. When mixing the powder with food (not more than a few spoonfuls), be careful to get all of it, avoid inhaling the powder (which could cause a reaction), and clean up afterward.
- Review dosing and management of unused doses with your doctor. I suggest bringing unused doses to up-dosing visits for review.
- Do not exercise or take a hot bath or shower for three hours after taking the dose. Don't take the dose after exercise or a hot shower or bath until after a cool-down period.
- Take the dose around the same time each day, with a meal, preferably dinner.
- Be around people familiar with this process; reactions typically occur within an hour of dosing but could occur hours later.
- Don't dose if you are going for an up-dose visit the same day.
- NEVER take more than the daily dose. If you missed days, let your doctor know. It could be dangerous to try to double-up, for example.

In some cases, dosing may need to be resumed under direct medical supervision.

- There are a variety of conditions (what are called augmentation factors; see chapter 4) that can make someone more susceptible to an allergic reaction to an allergen, including a previously tolerated dose of OIT. These include fever/infections, exercise, ingesting alcohol, menstruation, using products containing aspirin or ibuprofen, and being stressed or tired. These should be watched out for and discussed with your doctor. Your doctor may have you skip some days of dosing during an illness. If aspirin or ibuprofen is needed, consideration should be given for administering it at a different time of the day and not around the time of OIT dosing.
- Let your doctor know about reactions or concerns.

Who is a good candidate for Palforzia?

Deciding upon this therapy requires careful consideration by you and your allergist. The buzzwords are "shared decision-making," meaning a conversation. OIT is a process, and it is not for everyone. The child must understand the purpose and limitations. The family must understand the burdens, costs (time and money), and possible outcomes. There is a trade-off of taking on the process of OIT to raise threshold of reaction against the possible side effects involved. The therapy has been considered somewhat controversial because it typically induces more allergic reactions than avoidance. While there is some controversy, OIT likely improves quality of life for many, reducing anxiety, and reduces the risk of reaction from accidental exposure. This is not the case for all, however. Avoidance or waiting for alternative future therapies may be preferred. Everyone involved must understand that this is a treatment, not a cure. It is a long-term commitment, and avoidance and preparation to treat a reaction continue. Of course, if the commitment is made to start, and the process becomes problematic or induces too many reactions, it can be discontinued (about 20% of the time, this seems to occur). Some features that may align with a good candidate:

- Understands what the therapy provides and does not provide (goals align with expectations of therapy)
- Motivated
- Sufficiently sensitive to peanut to warrant the procedure

- Having allergic reactions to accidental exposures despite care to avoid
- Detail oriented
- Able to recognize and willing to treat allergic reactions / anaphylaxis without hesitations about using epinephrine
- Able to devote time and effort
- Costs are manageable
- Everyone's best interest is being served
- Approach seems likely to improve quality of life and/or anxiety for the individual rather than increase it
- Family and patient are aligned
- Ready for a long-term commitment

Who is not a good candidate for Palforzia?

Some people may not be interested in this approach. They may have gone for many years with no reactions, are not feeling overly restricted by the allergy, and consider the process of OIT a burden. Many may weigh the risks and benefits and prefer avoidance. Some may find the approach more anxiety-provoking than avoidance. Families may benefit from discussing the treatment not only with their allergist, but also with a mental health professional.

Some may not be very sensitive to peanut in the first place. The studies on Palforzia excluded people who tolerated the 100-milligram dose of peanut, which in feeding tests follows smaller doses accumulating to about half of a peanut. The Palforzia studies also selected those with strongly positive peanut blood (>15 kU/L) or skin tests (>8 millimeters) deemed more likely to be very sensitive to small amounts (although this is not often the case). Many people (almost half with a peanut allergy) can already consume the final dose of 300-milligram Palforzia, or more, with no or mild symptoms, and so dedicating the time to this therapy would seem unnecessary. There are no simple tests to predict threshold, but this should be considered prior to embarking on the therapy.

Having strong test results or prior severe reactions to trace exposures is NOT a reason to discount therapy, although the rate of side effects may be higher and chance of success lower than average.

There are specific problems that are considered "contraindications." Some features that may suggest a person may not be, at least not currently, a good candidate:

- Not confirmed to have a peanut allergy
- Patient or family not strongly motivated to pursue the therapy
- Has uncontrolled asthma
- Eosinophilic esophagitis or other eosinophilic gut diseases (evaluate if there is a history of trouble swallowing, pain with eating, vomiting, heartburn, or reflux)
- Circumstances or disposition making it difficult to commit to the necessary routine or rules
- Not very sensitive to peanut
- Does not see the benefit of raising threshold and bearing with the time and possible side effects compared to continued avoidance
- Unable to commit the time or resources
- Need to take medications that could reduce effectiveness or interfere with epinephrine (such as beta blockers) or heart problems that make anaphylaxis more risky
- Pregnant
- Reluctant to use self-injectable epinephrine
- Unable to allocate a daily three-hour period with no exercise

What is the long-term outcome of being on Palforzia? When do I stop?
From the studies that we have thus far, it appears that discontinuation of therapy will result in loss of protection over time. The loss of protection does not happen immediately and can be expected to vary by person and the length of time on therapy (slower loss for longer time on treatment). When my patients ask, "Do I have to take this for the rest of my life?" I answer that the therapy has to be continued "indefinitely," but it is hard for me to imagine that they would not eventually be switching to a better, easier, or more definitive therapy. Yet long-term studies are not available, and perhaps over many, many years a more permanent effect does take hold. Admittedly, however, studies in adults thus far were not as definitive as children, and we don't really know the outcomes for people who start in childhood and continue into adulthood.

Importantly, Palforzia aims for a convenient daily dose that raises the threshold for most, well above a level typical of small accidental exposures. Studies on peanut OIT have also aimed for higher maintenance doses, including daily meal-sized amounts. A strategy toward a higher dose of peanut could result in including peanut as a routine part of the diet, rather than a daily dose, which some may prefer. Others may have aversions to peanut and would not prefer this approach. In the limited studies of high-dose treatment, long periods of abstinence can still result in loss of protection. Palforzia is a new therapy, and transitioning people from Palforzia to higher amounts of peanut is something that will be explored. My research group is currently studying whether people who are already "bite safe" to peanut and would not be good candidates for Palforzia, as they already tolerate modest amounts of peanut, are better off simply continuing avoidance (since they are not at high risk from small exposures) or are better off pushing to much higher amounts to try to include peanut as a routine part of the diet in meal-sized amounts. We hope to understand this better in the coming years.

Is there a best age to start Palforzia or peanut OIT? Younger? Teenage?
Currently, Palforzia is approved from age 4 years, but studies in younger children and infants are underway. Preliminary studies suggest that younger children/infants may be more amenable to the therapy and may even have a more permanent response. Giving this therapy to infants and toddlers is tricky, as they cannot voice their symptoms.

Many parents want to start Palforzia for their teenagers because they are worried about the independence of high school and college. This is an understandable view. For this age group, I think it is particularly important to make sure the young adult understands the risks, benefits, and the limitations of the approach. We must depend upon them to take the daily dose religiously, follow the rules (daily dosing, no exercise, avoid alcohol, etc.), continue to avoid peanut, and be willing to treat an allergic reaction to the treatment independently.

Should I use Palforzia or just grocery store peanut?
A benefit of Palforzia is that the doses are carefully crafted, measured, and safe from contamination. Risks and benefits have been carefully delineated from monitored studies. Answers to the questions below will address using "grocery store" foods for OIT, but increasing numbers of allergy practices have used store-bought peanut, measuring and diluting doses in-house. A survey found that most allergists are more comfortable using an FDA-approved product (see Greenhawt and Vickery in chapter 11). The impact of switching from the "top dose" or Palforzia to some real-food equivalent (such as a peanut or small amount of peanut butter) has not yet been investigated, but as mentioned above, some studies have aimed for doses higher than 300 milligrams.

Indeed, many studies have transitioned people who are on high doses of OIT to use "real food" equivalents. For example, instead of taking a dose of powder, real food is eaten. In our study of egg oral immunotherapy, as one example, we aimed for a top daily dose of the equivalent of one-third of one egg. If the child could eat more than one egg after that treatment, and kept that threshold after about five weeks without dosing, we advised them to add egg to the diet. For those who did not get there but were on the treatment, we let them work out a plan with their allergist to trial regular egg products. There was a five-year follow-up period after the study ended (see Kim et al. in chapter 11). We found that most of the children were eating bakery foods with egg, and about two-thirds were eating regular egg. Indeed, for foods like egg, milk, and wheat, studies on OIT have often aimed for much higher doses, with the intention to liberalize ingestion of the food toward "free eating" or "real food" equivalents.

What is the status of OIT for foods other than peanut?

Peanut is the first target of a pharmaceutical form of OIT treatment. As indicated above, the path has been controversial. Health care agencies worry that the treatment overall results in more reactions than avoidance, but they have likely underestimated potential positive impact on quality of life. Meanwhile, many foods have been investigated, including egg, milk, sesame, various tree nuts, wheat, and others. OIT to multiple foods at the same time has also been investigated (see Otani et al. in chapter 11). Although the approach to foods other than peanut is generally the same, giving a gradual increase in dose over time, there are likely nuances that cause variations on outcomes. Still, a majority of people in most studies can be desensitized. Without extensive monitored studies, however, and without carefully reviewed protocols, the outcomes are harder to delineate.

How do I get OIT for foods other than peanut?

The use of OIT is gaining increasing acceptance, despite the aforementioned controversy. As noted above, the details regarding peanut alone are complex. Safety and efficacy are not fully understood, practical considerations abound, and protocols vary. In their review of peanut OIT, the Institute for Clinical and Economic Research (ICER) in 2019 reviewed the evidence and asked the question, "Is the evidence adequate to demonstrate that the net health benefit of [Palforzia] plus strict peanut avoidance is superior to continued avoidance alone?" In response, 12 out of 16 members voted no. Approaching OIT for other foods or multiple foods adds additional layers of complexity over the FDA-approved peanut OIT. In the United States, OIT is offered by a minority of allergists. It is being studied in many research centers. Most practicing allergists have been hoping for FDA-approved treatments. A study is currently ongoing to evaluate a mixture of foods used for OIT.

Why aren't all foods FDA approved for OIT?

Foods used for treating food allergy fit the FDA definition of a drug. Indeed, they pose risks and potential benefits. FDA-approved products for OIT, like Palforzia, would be carefully studied, have specific risks and benefits delineated, are monitored carefully, and the product itself would need to fulfill specifications regarding protein content, consistency, and safety (for example, monitoring bacterial and toxin contamination). Studies suggest, for example, that different off-the-shelf peanut products have different ratios of peanut allergens. These circumstances have resulted in controversy. Given that OIT can induce anaphylaxis, does it make sense to offer this therapy with off-the-shelf foods and various, possibly personalized, protocols? Can patients rely on their local allergist to administer the treatments safely without additional guidance? How do patients assess safety and effectiveness when a "home brew" approach is being used? Conversely, evidence is mounting from increasing studies, but FDA approval would likely take years for each food. For many foods, some protocols have been vetted in studies. Are they "ready for prime time" without further study?

What is the current thinking about OIT for foods other than peanut?

US guidelines from 2010 and 2014 advised against OIT. As the number of published studies increased, a 2018 European guideline noted the important risks and benefits and concluded that OIT should "only be performed in research centers or in clinical centers with an extensive experience." In 2020, the Canadian Society for Allergy and Clinical Immunology published a broad set of recommendations derived from literature reviews and stakeholder deliberations (see Bégin et al. in chapter 11). These guidelines acknowledge the promise but also the costs, limitations, ethical and safety issues, and unknowns of OIT, essentially recommending the approach but suggesting that a shared responsibility among stakeholders is needed. In 2020, the lay organization Food Allergy Research & Education (FARE) published a report from a summit on OIT that convened various stakeholders (see Pepper et al. in chapter 11). This summit resulted in a number of con-clusions, many of them aligned with the information discussed previously about Palforzia. Some conclusions are summarized as follows:

- OIT is an emerging option.
- OIT is not appropriate for all food-allergic patients. Shared decision-making is needed.
- Patients considered as candidates for OIT must have confirmed IgE mediated food allergy.
- OIT may not be appropriate for patients with a high likelihood to out-grow the allergy.
- OIT is most beneficial for informed, motivated patients and families who seek enhanced normalcy and accept the added risks and burdens of treatment.
- Practices offering OIT should be competent in the diagnosis of food allergy, administration of oral food challenges, and the management of anaphylaxis. OIT should be performed under the supervision of a board-certified allergist.
- The possible goals ("bite safe" versus "eating") and outcomes (chance of success, burdens, reactions) and approach (regimen) should be dis-cussed and clarified, although more research is needed in this area.
- Asthma and allergic diseases should be well controlled.
- Providing OIT to people with EoE should be avoided.
- The psychosocial impact of food allergy and OIT should be explored with mental health services as needed.
- If non-FDA-approved products are used, this should be communicated clearly, including risk of adverse events. Any product should have clearly labeled protein content and risk of cross-contamination, and should be continuously monitored for consistency.
- Financial costs should be discussed.
- Social and family dynamics should be evaluated.
- Restrictions on exercise and other activities should be discussed to evaluate OIT fit to lifestyle.

The FARE summit also identified "unmet needs" for OIT, including improved measures on the impact of OIT on health and well-being, better understanding of safety and effectiveness, identification of optimal dosing, more understanding of approaching multiple foods at one time, identifica-tion as to whether OIT reduces allergic reaction rates, and comparisons of FDA-approved versus shelf-bought products used for OIT.

What should I look out for if pursuing OIT outside of clinical studies, or with non-FDA-approved products?

OIT is an exciting and promising approach, but it is not without risks, costs, and burdens. Currently, few allergists offer this treatment. Many allergists are interested in starting programs, and some commercial entities specifically focused on OIT are also forming. Information on OIT has come a long way in a short time, but more study is needed. The fast movement from clinical trials to clinical practice means that there will be unknowns. I have been concerned to see some allergy practices that in the past did not offer oral food challenges, owing to worries about having allergic reactions in their offices, now perform OIT. I think that practices who undertake OIT should be comfortable diagnosing food allergy with food challenges and managing allergic reactions. Importantly, some clinical practices have been publishing their "real-world" experience with OIT (see Wasserman et al. and Afinogenova et al. in chapter 11). Although the tracking of effectiveness and side effects is typically less rigorous in these publications compared to regulated clinical trials, many of these reports for peanut OIT align with those from clinical trials, with similar rates of "success" and dropout (about 20%) as the Palforzia studies. This observation is telling. If a practice is advertising unusually high success rates, one may wonder what they are counting as success or if they are selecting patients who are not particularly allergic.

In summary, the interested patient must proceed with caution and take a buyer-beware approach. Are you comfortable with the allergist and staff? Are you comfortable with therapies that are not approved or regulated by the FDA? Are the practices providing information about their experience, the protocols they are using, and the details about products they are using? Have they explained why you or your child is a candidate for the treatment? Do they have safety in mind? Have you had all of your questions answered? Is the "fit" right for you and your family?

What alternatives are there to OIT?

The default alternative is to avoid the food. As described above, OIT is associated with allergic reactions, and it carries risks and burdens. OIT is not for everyone. Avoidance is perfectly acceptable and still the usual approach. It is also OK to take a wait-and-see approach. OIT is still in its early stages, and many want to see how the FDA-approved product's use unfolds. Additional therapies are in the pipeline as well, and clinical trials can also be considered.

What are the advantages or disadvantages of oral versus sublingual immunotherapy for food allergies?

From studies available thus far, it appears that the oral route of treatment, compared to the sublingual, is more effective but also more likely to cause allergic reactions.

If a person with milk or egg allergies can tolerate eating these foods when they are baked into breads or muffins, does eating these foods help to treat these allergies?

As discussed in chapter 6, about 70% to 80% of children with allergy to whole forms of milk or eggs (scrambled eggs, French toast, cheese, ice cream, and so on) can tolerate baked goods with these ingredients. Some studies of milk and eggs have suggested that the milk- or egg-allergic children who tolerate these extensively heated foods and go ahead and eat them show immune changes that are similar to those of people treated with oral or sublingual immunotherapy, and that this may speed recovery compared with strict avoidance, although the evidence is mixed (see Upton and Nowak-Wegrzyn in chapter 11).

What is epicutaneous (on the skin) immunotherapy for food allergy?

Another approach to immunotherapy is to expose immune cells in the skin to the food. The theory is that immune cells in the skin may promote a nonallergic response to the food over time. A drug company has created a skin patch to slowly deliver food protein into the skin. The product aimed to treat peanut allergy is called Viaskin Peanut. The company has milk and egg patches also under development and study.

What are advantages of epicutaneous immunotherapy for food allergy?

A primary advantage of epicutaneous immunotherapy (EPIT) is safety, because exposing the skin to the food protein is unlikely to trigger anaphylaxis, although rashes are common. Unlike the oral or sublingual therapies, there are essentially no gut symptoms, and allergic reactions beyond the patch location and anaphylaxis are uncommon.

How effective is EPIT for food allergies?

Preliminary studies looked at a large age range, but children older than 11 years of age who started the treatment did not appear to receive any benefit. A study was conducted of 356 children ages 4 to 11 years who were reactive at a dose of 300 milligrams of peanut or less (Fleischer et al. 2019; see chapter 11). Success was defined as tolerating a 300-milligram dose for those who had reacted at 10 milligrams or less, and tolerating a 1,000-milligram dose for the remainder. The study found that 35.3% treated met that response, compared to 13.6% on placebo. Another way of looking at it was that about 50% improved from reacting at less than one-third of a peanut to being able to have one peanut or more before reacting (this was the case for 19% on placebo). In open treatment studies, an additional two years of therapy continued to show improvement (Fleischer et al. 2020; see chapter 11). About half of those who completed three years of therapy were able to eat a 1,000-milligram dose or more, compared to 40% of this group at the end of the first year, and 76% had improved from baseline. In summary, the treatment was not as robust as that seen with, for example, OIT, but the side effect profile is favorable.

What is the status of the peanut patch or other food patches?

As of 2021, studies continue, and there are hopes of FDA approval.

How do you know if OIT, SLIT, or EPIT is "working"?

As noted from the information above, studies of these therapies rely upon oral food challenges. Many people who tried to enroll in studies of these therapies were denied entry because they were not allergic enough to qualify (they tolerated too much peanut in their oral food challenge at the start of the study). A big question for using these therapies is identifying people who are sensitive enough to need them. Once under treatment, the food challenge can show if the therapy is working. Without a food challenge, we are only assuming the effectiveness for an individual. Studies are trying to identify "biomarkers" or tests that could show effect without undertaking an oral food challenge. In the meantime, without a feeding test, effectiveness is being assumed. This is most clearly the case for SLIT and EPIT. In contrast, with OIT, the side effects, or lack of them, may at least give some feedback on whether progress is being made.

Is there a potential for combining therapies?

Yes. For example, low doses of a food given by SLIT or EPIT may be a starting point for using larger doses in oral immunotherapy. Also, using anti-IgE therapy prior to and while initially increasing doses of oral immunotherapy may potentially reduce side effects and improve the effectiveness of the treatment. Studies are also looking at using OIT with dupilumab (to try to reduce side effects and improve efficacy) or even combining anti-IgE and dupilumab.

What is the progress in using immunotherapy and anti-IgE treatment at the same time for food allergies?

Several studies have looked at this combination. The rationale is to start oral immunotherapy after a period of treatment with anti-IgE injections, since these injections should improve the threshold of allergic reactions to the oral immunotherapy (see Nadeau et al. in chapter 11). After a person is on the final daily doses of the oral immunotherapy, the anti-IgE treatment could be discontinued. Initial studies have been promising in perhaps reducing, although not eliminating, the reactions to dosing. Children have typically been able to progress faster to higher amounts of one or even several (simultaneously) food allergens while being given anti-IgE injections, compared to using the oral immunotherapy without anti-IgE injections (see Wood et al. in chapter 11). The anti-IgE treatment has not reduced stomach symptoms as much as it has reduced hives and anaphylaxis. It does not seem to reduce the risk of developing eosinophilic esophagitis or of making the oral immunotherapy more likely to result in persistent protection if the oral immunotherapy is stopped. However, many more children tolerate the oral immunotherapy with fewer symptoms when on the injections. More studies are underway to better understand the promise of this approach. One such study is called OUTMATCH, with results expected by 2024.

What additional treatments are being evaluated to treat food allergies?

See chapter 11 to learn more about how to access information on current studies. Some novel therapies that were promising in preclinical studies may be ready for trials in people, and many are already in initial safety studies. It is almost certain that treatments that are an improvement over OIT or are better suited to specific people with food allergies will become available in the coming years.

Treatments of Specific Food-Allergic Diseases

What treatments are being evaluated for eosinophilic esophagitis?
Current treatments include dietary avoidance of allergens and use of steroids. New therapies are targeting the cells and chemicals that direct the allergic inflammation. See chapter 5 for more information about this illness and its treatment.

What treatments are being evaluated to treat anaphylaxis?
New forms of epinephrine autoinjectors are being considered. Drugs and other treatments to block the cells and chemicals that cause the symptoms are being analyzed.

What treatments are being evaluated to treat oral allergy syndrome?
Allergen immunotherapy (allergy shots) and other treatments of pollen allergy may have the useful additional benefit of also reducing or eliminating symptoms from the food proteins that are similar to the pollen proteins.

What treatments are being tested for food protein–induced enterocolitis syndrome?
Currently, the main therapy for FPIES is food avoidance. Studies are attempting to determine the cells and immune responses that are causing these reactions so that targets for treatments can be found. It is not currently known whether treatments for IgE-mediated allergy, such as oral immunotherapy, or EPIT would help enterocolitis syndrome, but studies are beginning to look at this possibility.

Unproven Treatments

What food allergy treatments are unproven?
Throughout this book, various approaches to treatment are discussed that remain under study and may be considered "unproven," or perhaps only partly proven. This is a somewhat semantic concern. For example, oral immunotherapy has been shown to alter the threshold of reactivity to foods

for many people, and so in one way it has been proven to work, yet more needs to be done to determine whether the effects can be long-lasting as well as to minimize side effects. So, oral immunotherapy could be considered partly unproven. Other treatments, however, would be considered inappropriate because they are unproven or even disproven and not based on firm evidence.

What food allergy treatments would be considered inappropriate?

Traditional allergists consider several approaches used today to be inappropriate. These include acupressure, chiropractic manipulation, provocation-neutralization therapy, rotation diets, orthomolecular therapy, mercury amalgam removal, urine autoinjection, laser therapy, antifungal therapy, and immune system–boosting elimination diets.

What is provocation-neutralization therapy?

This treatment, also discussed in chapter 3, relies on diagnosing food allergies by provoking symptoms using dilutions of the allergen and then treating them by using a weaker "neutralizing" dose. The treatment has been disproven in well-designed studies.

What are rotation diets?

The general theory is that there may be foods in the diet causing "symptoms," and by rotating what is eaten every four or five days, the body is not exposed to large amounts of any particular problematic food. Additionally, the theory is that reducing continued exposure to certain foods would reduce the chance of developing problems with them. This theory runs counter to many proven aspects of food allergy; for example, if a food is an allergen for a person, symptoms will arise whenever the food is eaten. It is also counter to the observation that maintaining exposure to a food may actually reduce the chance of allergy in some cases.

What is orthomolecular therapy?

This treatment approach, used infrequently for food allergy but often for a variety of maladies, relies on giving large doses of various vitamins, supplements, and antioxidants in response to measurement of vitamins in the serum. There are no controlled studies of this approach, and there are dangers of overdosing vitamins.

What is mercury amalgam removal?

There is a theory that silver-mercury amalgam used in dental fillings may cause sensitivity that results in various maladies and symptoms. This theory remains unproven, so removal of the fillings as a treatment is unproven.

What is urine autoinjection?

Based on observations in the 1930s that the urine of some allergic people injected into their own skin caused a response but that their urine injected into another person did not, some practitioners began to inject urine as a treatment of various illnesses (allergies, stomach complaints, jaundice, and so forth). There were never any good studies on the effectiveness, and this treatment could actually promote adverse immune responses against the body's own proteins. Professional organizations have warned against this practice as being unproven, without scientific basis, and potentially dangerous.

What is laser therapy?

The laser method purportedly uses a biofeedback machine to simulate and test reactions to thousands of allergens before a laser is used to stimulate the nervous system. No studies support the claim that this technology cures allergies. Some advertise that the approach is FDA approved, which is not accurate.

What is antifungal therapy?

There is a theory that yeast in the body, Candida, is responsible for a "yeast hypersensitivity syndrome" in which overgrowth results in inflammation and toxins. The symptoms attributed to this include fatigue, heartburn, bloating, diarrhea, constipation, depression, and memory problems. Candida and other fungi are normal inhabitants of the body, however, and there is no routine diagnostic approach to an overgrowth or toxic effect. Treatments have included various diets and antifungal therapies. A scientific basis for a syndrome has never been established. One well-controlled study did not show improvement in general symptoms of fatigue or depression from treatments against the fungus.

What are immune system–boosting elimination diets?

Through combinations of testing and using traditional or alternative and unproven methods, numerous foods are eliminated from the diet to treat presumed "multiple food allergy," with the notion that doing so may improve the immune system. Often, the person is given various dietary supplements. There is no evidence that removing multiple foods improves immune function, and doing so may increase the risk of problems from malnutrition.

Participating in Food Allergy Research

What is it like to participate in food allergy clinical trials?

Most clinical trials of food allergy involve a screening visit to ensure that the participant is otherwise generally healthy and qualifies for the study. An initial feeding test is often used to determine how much food can be consumed before symptoms occur. Next, treatment is started (randomized, like a coin toss, to receive the therapy being tested or placebo), and after some period another feeding test is performed to check for effectiveness, comparing the treatment to placebo. During the entire study, the participant keeps in close contact with the study investigators and staff.

Should I participate in clinical trials for food allergy?

This is a personal decision. If people did not participate, however, we would never learn whether a treatment works, and no progress would be made. In fact, recruitment of participants into research studies—for all treatments, not just food allergy—is a major hurdle that results in delays in moving treatments forward or in learning which ones to abandon. If a clinical trial is not for you, you can still contribute to food allergy research by participating in studies that involve only questionnaires or a blood sample, through donations toward research, or through advocacy.

What are the advantages of participating in clinical trials for food allergy?

The primary advantage is to help determine whether a particular approach is viable for treating food allergy. There is a potential benefit for the participant to experience some improvement in the allergy, but if this were a definite benefit, there would be no need for a study! Participants often feel empowered because they are doing something to help themselves and others who are suffering with food allergies (whether or not the treatment under study is proven effective).

What are the disadvantages of participating in clinical trials for food allergy?

There are some general risks associated with trying a new therapy because there may be side effects. These would be described in detail and would depend on the approach and type of study. Other disadvantages are related to time commitments and discomfort (such as blood tests). These issues vary greatly among studies. Most treatment trials are mimicking what would be done should the therapy prove to be effective. Thus the number of visits is not much different from what would be done if the therapy became routine clinical practice.

What is done to ensure safety if I participate in clinical trials for food allergy?

Many things. Investigators are likely to explain that they would not enroll people into a trial unless they would have themselves or their own family members participate as well. As described earlier in this chapter, the study procedures are evaluated by external reviewers, often through numerous different regulators. Each procedure is performed under appropriate supervision to ensure safety. Any adverse effects are monitored and evaluated. Privacy is as carefully protected as possible under law. And participants are always free to leave a study at any time. In fact, if the investigators are concerned about a participant's safety, they can remove the person from the study, even if the participant wanted to continue.

How are people selected for clinical trials of food allergy?

The entry criteria for a study typically address the illness being studied. For example, a study of a treatment for milk allergy requires people with milk allergy. Depending on several factors, an age range may be specified.

Why are some people excluded from clinical trials of food allergy?

All studies establish criteria that exclude participants. Sometimes the exclusions have to do with the treatment being used. For example, a person who makes too much or no IgE may not qualify for a study of an anti-IgE therapy. Often, people cannot participate if they are on treatments that might interfere with evaluating the response to the therapy being tested. Many of the exclusions are for safety reasons; for example, a person with significant medical problems other than food allergy is not likely to be a good candidate because there could be added risks arising from those health issues. The same is true for having severe, poorly controlled asthma.

Why are specific age groups included in individual studies for food allergy treatments?

When treatments are initially trialed, healthy adults may be the first to be tested, so that the researchers can learn how the body manages the treatment. As therapies are tested further, adults, teenagers, or children over age 12 might be tested initially before trying the therapy on younger children— again, to ensure safety. Also, the older participants are better able to discuss any side effects.

Should I be concerned about the oral food challenges that are part of food allergy trials?

Oral food challenges are discussed in detail in chapter 3. When they are performed in research studies, the risk of having symptoms is greater because, unlike diagnostic tests, the person being tested is assumed to be allergic. Therefore starting doses and timing of doses are likely to be different in research studies. Still, the purpose of the feeding test is to determine how much of the food triggers symptoms; the purpose is *not to cause a severe reaction*. The feeding is stopped when a reaction is evident. The most common symptoms are skin and gut symptoms. The studies are always performed under medical supervision. Discuss any concerns with your study doctor.

What if I am randomly assigned to the placebo in a food allergy clinical trial?

Potential research participants may feel that they do not want to participate because they do not want to be randomized to receive the placebo. There are many reasons this should not be a concern:

• The study is not likely to be valid if there is no placebo comparison. In a study of anti-IgE therapy, the placebo group was able to eat three times more peanuts after therapy (placebo therapy). This sounds pretty good, but any ineffective treatment could have this placebo effect. If you participate in a study without a placebo group, the chance that the study will provide strong evidence for or against the new therapy is diminished, and your commitment may not have been as worthwhile in finding an answer.

- If the therapy does work, and you were in the placebo group, you will still have access, eventually, to a useful treatment.
- If the therapy had unanticipated side effects, you will have avoided them.

How do I find out about clinical trials and food allergy?

There are many sources (see chapter 11). In the United States, an excellent resource is www.clinicaltrials.gov, where you can search for clinical trials using terms that describe what you are looking for (for example, milk allergy).

How do I stay informed about new treatments for food allergy?

Get on a mailing list of any nearby research centers, join lay organizations and support groups, and visit the websites that act as clearinghouses for trials and for other types of food allergy research.

How do I become an advocate for food allergy research?

Join a group! See the resources in chapter 11.

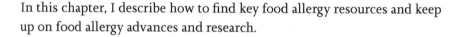

CHAPTER 11

Accessing Help and Information to Manage Food Allergies

In this chapter, I describe how to find key food allergy resources and keep up on food allergy advances and research.

Educational Resources

What should I do to learn more about managing my food allergies?
You made great progress by reading this book. But for additional education, start with your allergist. Make lists of questions to discuss at your next visit. Find out whether other specialists (dietitian, gastroenterologist, counselor, and so on) would be useful to consult. Check the Internet for websites, books, support groups, and organizations.

What types of resources are available for managing life with food allergies?
There are numerous resources. It would take up an entire book just to list them. The following chart shows what is out there in a general sense, so you can access or find these resources through the Internet.

Resources for Managing Life with Food Allergies

Websites
General information about food allergies, specific food allergies (e.g., peanut), professional societies, government agencies, foundations, sites for children, manufacturers catering to food allergy, pharmaceutical companies (emergency medications), blogs, chat rooms

Books, videos, and magazines
These resources cover virtually every topic, including ones focused on management for children, parents, educators; those that are food specific (such as about milk, peanuts, tree nuts); psychological issues; advice from people living with food allergies; cookbooks; and lifestyle publications.

Apps
Emergency information, allergy management

Foods
Allergen-free specialty manufacturers; local allergy-friendly restaurants and bakeries; cookbooks; recipes

Gadgets and practical materials
Carrying cases for medications, allergen labels, examples of allergy-related school forms, medical identification jewelry

Awareness products
Clothing, stuffed animals, jewelry, wristbands, gifts

How do I know what resources to trust?
Unfortunately, individuals and organizations may provide advice or services that are not necessarily based on good evidence. This is a buyer-beware situation. When it seems too good to be true, it probably is. Consider the source. Is there recognized expertise? Is there external review? For organizations, is there a medical advisory board (there should be), and who are the members? For services, is there a track record? I suggest taking special caution in reviewing chat rooms and message boards that are not monitored. Sometimes

poor or inaccurate advice is dispensed by persons who are not experts in food allergies.

What websites should I use?

The good news about food allergy education and resources is that there has been an explosion of Internet resources. These include the websites of major lay and professional organizations as well as small groups with specific interests in particular food-related illnesses. There are websites dedicated to specific allergies, preparing meals, eating at restaurants and schools, cooking for persons on restricted diets, and many other topics. There are countless international resources and numerous blogs. It is not feasible to list all the potential resources, but I have included here some key websites that can also form the basis of a gateway to other resources. The list is clearly not exhaustive, and most of the resources I listed are government agencies, professional societies, and nonprofit organizations.

Selected Internet Resources on Food Allergies

Food Allergy Research & Education (FARE)
www.foodallergy.org

This lay organization partners with many international groups to address all areas of interest in food allergy and anaphylaxis, emphasizing research, education, and advocacy. The website is an excellent gateway to resources.

National Institute of Allergy and Infectious Diseases:
Food Allergy Guidelines and Peanut Prevention Addendum

Guidelines for the Diagnosis and Management of Food Allergies in the United States:
https://www.niaid.nih.gov/sites/default/files/faguidelinespatient.pdf

Addendum Guidelines for the Prevention of Peanut Allergy in the United States:
https://www.niaid.nih.gov/sites/default/files/peanut-allergy-prevention
-guidelines-parent-summary.pdf

The US Food and Drug Administration and Its Center for Food Safety and Applied Nutrition
www.fda.gov/food

The FDA provides a comprehensive listing of useful information about government-related notifications on food safety and allergen issues.

Centers for Disease Control: Food Allergies in Schools
www.cdc.gov/healthyschools/foodallergies

Learn more about CDC educational materials and initiatives related to food allergies in schools.

The International FPIES Association
www.fpies.org

The FPIES Foundation
www.fpiesfoundation.org

These are the websites of two lay organizations focused on food protein–induced enterocolitis syndrome.

American Partnership for Eosinophilic Disorders
http://apfed.org

This lay organization focuses on eosinophilic disorders, such as eosinophilic esophagitis.

AllergyHome.org
www.allergyhome.org

Kids with Food Allergies Foundation
www.kidswithfoodallergies.org

Families and caregivers of children with food allergies can find support and educational resources on these websites.

National Eczema Assocsiation
www.nationaleczema.org

Coalition of Skin Diseases
www.coalitionofskindiseases.org

These lay organizations focusing on allergic skin diseases provide multiple resources for information and support.

Asthma and Allergy Network
www.allergyasthmanetwork.org

Asthma and Allergy Foundation of America
www.aafa.org
Focusing on asthma and allergies, these lay organizations offer resources and support.

Jaffe Food Allergy Institute at Mount Sinai
https://icahn.mssm.edu/research/jaffe

At the author's institutional homepage, you will find updates on research and clinical care.

ClinicalTrials.gov
www.clinicaltrials.gov

Learn about ongoing research studies and how you can participate in food allergy research. Search according to your interests, such as "food allergy" or "peanut allergy."

American Academy of Allergy, Asthma, and Immunology
www.aaaai.org

A professional medical organization, the AAAAI provides resources for the public as well.

American College of Allergy, Asthma, and Immunology
www.acaai.org

This site is home of another professional medical organization with resources for the public.

Mothers of Children Having Allergies
www.mochallergies.org

This group from Chicago aims to help parents by providing information and resources.

American Academy of Pediatrics
www.aap.org

This well-known professional medical organization has extensive pediatric resources.

Academy of Nutrition and Dietetics
www.eatright.org

Here you'll find information on nutritional issues from a professional organization of dietitians.

MedicAlert
www.medicalert.org

MedicAlert is a standard resource for obtaining medical identification jewelry.

Food Allergy Canada
www.foodallergycanada.ca

Anaphylaxis Campaign (UK)
www.anaphylaxis.org.uk

World Allergy Organization
www.worldallergy.org

Worldwide, there are numerous lay and professional organizations focusing on food allergy and anaphylaxis.

Is there an app for food allergy?

There are many, and the number continues to grow. You can find apps that scan bar codes and relay food allergen information, present information about related foods, track symptoms and diet, and provide interactive recipes. I encourage you to explore the increasing variety of apps for food allergy, but use caution. Two studies in 2015 and 2020 of food allergy apps found many limitations, with incomplete or erroneous information or poorly working products, especially among apps meant to scan bar codes for allergenic ingredients. Some apps are not based on medical evidence regarding food allergies. For example, botanically related foods are not necessarily all off-limits to a person allergic to one from a related group, as one app claims. Some apps provide restaurant food ingredients, but I urge caution. Discuss each meal separately with staff, and do not rely solely on an app. Some of the apps are based on notions of symptom relationships to foods that are unproven (for example, some behavioral aspects, fatigue, and so forth). Keeping apps up to date is also an issue, so it is important to double-check ingredient labels when following advice on shopping from an app.

What should I do to educate my allergic child about food allergies?

Again, start with your allergist for specific information. It is okay to ask your allergist, "Can you explain more about the allergy to my child?" There are books, websites, and programs specifically aimed toward children. A good place to begin is at www.foodallergy.org. The site has links to programs, newsletters, activities, and books for children and teenagers.

What can I do to educate my family about food allergies?

Sharing resources that you found to be helpful is a great start. Bring interested relatives to an allergist visit as well. There are books designed to introduce siblings and relatives to the basics of food allergy.

What should I do to educate others about food allergies?

Usually, a health care provider at a school or camp will be responsible for staff education. If there has not already been progress, however, you may wish to make that person aware of educational programs. New online programs with interactive educational features for teachers and others are available. Check www.foodallergy.org for the latest on these programs.

How can I educate schools or camps about food allergies?

You may wish to point them to the educational materials mentioned above and in chapter 6. One source is www.allergyready.com, which has interactive educational materials at no cost. Their How to C.A.R.E. for Students with Food Allergies online course has been developed in partnership with leading food allergy organizations and health care professionals to improve the quality of school personnel education. I reviewed this program and found it to be excellent.

Support Groups, Advocacy, and Research

What organizations provide laypersons with information about research, advocacy, and support?

There are many, but leading the charge in the United States is Food Allergy Research & Education (FARE).

Are there support groups for food allergies?

Yes, and you can search for them at https://www.foodallergy.org/living-food -allergies/join-community/find-support-group.

How would I start a support group on food allergies?

You might start by talking to your allergist and others in your community who are interested. FARE is another resource.

How can I learn about advocacy for food allergies?

Check www.foodallergy.org. Advocacy activities, led in part by lay organizations, have achieved improved allergen food labeling, increased government research grants, improved school programs, better access to epinephrine in an emergency, and more effective approaches to food allergies in restaurants. But there is still much to do, and you can help.

How can I learn about participating in research studies about food allergies?

Check out Food Allergy Research & Education and www.clinicaltrials.gov, as listed above.

Handy Forms

What types of form letters or plans should I obtain from my doctor?

The two most common forms are the travel letter and the emergency action plan (see chapter 4). Versions are available from www.foodallergy.org and www.aap.org. An example travel letter is shown here.

DATE
RE: [Name, Date of Birth]

To Whom It May Concern:

My patient, named above, suffers from a life-threatening food allergy. This is a severe allergy that makes it medically necessary to carry an antihistamine and self-injectable epinephrine. Epinephrine is pre-scribed by a licensed medical professional, and my patient needs to have this life-saving medication available at all times, including during travel. A food-allergic reaction can result in severe symptoms, and this medication is needed promptly. Please allow my patient to have the self-injectable epinephrine and additional medications (antihistamine and asthma medications, if needed) on board the airplane. Because of the food allergies, my patient may need to carry sufficient food as well.

Sincerely,

_____, MD

Cited Medical References and Additional Articles of Interest

Abrams EM, Chan ES, Sicherer S. Peanut allergy: new advances and ongo-ing controversies. Pediatrics. 2020;145:e20192102. doi:10.1542/peds .2019-2102.

Afinogenova Y, Rubin TN, Patel SD, Powell RL, et al. Community private practice clinical experience with peanut oral immunotherapy. J Allergy Clin Immunol Pract. 2020;8:2727–35.

Allen KJ, Turner PJ, Pawankar R, Taylor S, et al. Precautionary labelling of foods for allergen content: are we ready for a global framework? World Allergy Organ J. 2014;7:10. doi:10.1186/1939-4551-7-10.

Annunziato RA, Shemesh E, Weiss CC, Izzo GN, D'Urso C, Sicherer SH. An assessment of the mental health care needs and utilization by families of children with a food allergy. J Health Psychol. 2013;18:1456–64.

Ballmer-Weber BK, Fernandez-Rivas M, Beyer K, Deferenz M, et al. How much is too much? threshold dose distributions for 5 food allergens. J Allergy Clin Immunol. 2015;135:964–71.

Bartnikas LM, Huffaker MF, Sheehan WJ, Kanchongkittiphon W, et al. Impact of school peanut-free policies on epinephrine administration. J Allergy Clin Immunol. 2017;140:465–73.

Bégin P, Chan ES, Kim H, Wagner M, et al. CSACI guidelines for the ethical, evidence-based and patient-oriented clinical practice of oral immunotherapy in IgE-mediated food allergy. Allergy Asthma Clin Immunol. 2020 Mar 18;16:20. doi:10.1186/s13223-020-0413-7.

Boyce JA, Assa'ad A, Burks AW, Jones, SM, et al. Guidelines for the diagnosis and management of food allergy in the United States: report of the NIAID-sponsored expert panel. J Allergy Clin Immunol. 2010;126:S1-58.

Brough HA, Liu AH, Sicherer S, Makinson K, et al. Atopic dermatitis increases the effect of exposure to peanut antigen in dust on peanut sensitization and likely peanut allergy. J Allergy Clin Immunol. 2015;135:164–70.

Chang A, Robison R, Cai M, Singh AM. Natural history of food-triggered atopic dermatitis and development of immediate reactions in children. J Allergy Clin Immunol Pract. 2016;4:229–36.

Chinthrajah RS, Purington N, Andorf S, Long A, et al. Sustained outcomes in oral immunotherapy for peanut allergy (POISED study): a large, randomised, double-blind, placebo-controlled, phase 2 study. Lancet. 2019;394:1437–49.

Chu DK, Wood RA, French S, Fiocchi A, et al. Oral immunotherapy for peanut allergy (PACE): a systematic review and meta-analysis of efficacy and safety. Lancet. 2019;393:2222–32.

Committee on Food Allergies: Global Burden, Causes, Treatment, Prevention, and Public Policy, Food and Nutrition Board, Health and Medicine Division, National Academies of Sciences, Engineering and Medicine, Stallings VA, Oria M, eds. Finding a path to safety in food allergy: assessment of the global burden, causes, prevention, management, and public policy. National Academies Press, Washington, DC, 2016.

Cox AL, Eigenmann PA, Sicherer SH. Clinical relevance of cross-reactivity in food allergy. J Allergy Clin Immunol Pract. 2021;9:82–99.

de Silva D, Geromi M, Halken S, Host A, et al. Primary prevention of food allergy in children and adults: systematic review. Allergy. 2014;69: 581–89.

Du Toit G, Roberts G, Sayre PH, Bahnson HT, et al. Randomized trial of peanut consumption in infants at risk for peanut allergy. N Engl J Med. 2015;372:803–13.

Eigenmann PA, Sicherer SH, Borkowski TA, Cohen BA, Sampson HA. Prevalence of IgE-mediated food allergy among children with atopic dermatitis. Pediatrics. 1998;101:E8. doi:10.1542/peds.101.3.e8.

Eigenmann PA, Beyer K, Lack G, Muraro A, Ong PY, Sicherer SH, Sampson HA. Are avoidance diets still warranted in children with atopic dermatitis? Pediatr Allergy Immunol. 2019;31:19–26.

Fleischer DM, Perry TT, Atkins D, Wood RA, et al. Allergic reactions to foods in preschool-aged children in a prospective observational food allergy study. Pediatrics. 2012;130:e25-32. doi:10.1542/peds.2011-1762.

Fleischer DM, Greenhawt M, Sussman G, Begin P, et al. Effect of epicutaneous immunotherapy vs placebo on reaction to peanut protein ingestion among children with peanut allergy: the PEPITES Randomized Clinical Trial. JAMA. 2019;321:946–55.

Fleischer DM, Shreffler WG, Campbell DE, Green TD, et al. Long-term, open-label extension study of the efficacy and safety of epicutaneous immunotherapy for peanut allergy in children: PEOPLE 3-year results. J Allergy Clin Immunol. 2020;146:863–74.

Fleischer DM, Chan ES, Venter C, Spergel JM, et al. A consensus approach to primary prevention of food allergy through nutrition: guidance from the American Academy of Allergy, Asthma and Immunology; American College of Allergy, Asthma and Immunology; and the Canadian Society for Allergy and Clinical Immunology. J Allergy Clin Immunol Pract. 2021;9:22–43.

Foong R, Dantzer J, Wood RA, Santos AF. Improving diagnostic accuracy in food allergy. J Allergy Clin Immunol Pract 2021;9:71–80.

Ford LS, Taylor SL, Pacenza R, Niemann LM, Lambrecht DM, Sicherer SH. Food allergen advisory labeling and product contamination with egg, milk, and peanut. J Allergy Clin Immunol. 2010;126:384–85.

Franxman TJ, Howe L, Teich E, Greenhawt MJ. Oral food challenge and food allergy quality of life in caregivers of children with food allergy. J Allergy Clin Immunol Pract. 2015;3:50–56.

Greenhawt MJ, Vickery BP. Allergist-reported trends in the practice of food allergen oral immunotherapy. J Allergy Clin Immunol Pract. 2015;3:33–38.

Greer FR, Sicherer SH, Burks AW; Committee on Nutrition; Section on Allergy and Immunology. The effects of early nutritional interventions on the development of atopic disease in infants and children: the role of maternal dietary restriction, breastfeeding, hydrolyzed formulas, and timing of introduction of allergenic complementary foods. Pediatrics. 2019 Apr;143. pii:e20190281. doi:10.1542/peds.2019-0281.

Gupta RS, Walkner MM, Greenhawt M, Lau CH, et al. Food allergy sensitization and presentation in siblings of food allergic children. J Allergy Clin Immunol Pract. 2016;4:956–62.

Gupta RS, Warren CM, Smith BM, Blumenstock JA, et al. The public health impact of parent-reported childhood food allergies in the United States. Pediatrics. 2018:142:e20181235. doi:10.1542/peds.2018-1235.

Gupta RS, Warren CM, Smith BM, Jiang J, et al. Prevalence and severity of food allergies among US adults. JAMA Netw Open. 2019 Jan 4;2:e185630. doi:10.1001/jamanetworkopen.2018.5630.

Hefle SL, Furlong TJ, Niemann L, Lemon-Mule H, Sicherer S, Taylor SL. Consumer attitudes and risks associated with packaged foods having advisory labeling regarding the presence of peanuts. J Allergy Clin Immunol. 2007;120:171–76.

Herbert L, Shemesh E, Bender B. Clinical management of psychosocial concerns related to food allergy. J Allergy Clin Immunol Pract. 2016; 4:205–13.

Hill DA, Shuker M, Cianferoni A, Wong T, Ruchelli E, Spergel JM, Brown-Whitegorn TF. The development of IgE-mediated immediate hypersensitivity after the diagnosis of eosinophilic esophagitis to the same food. J Allergy Clin Immunol Pract. 2015;3:123–24.

Ho H-E, Chehade M. Development of IgE-mediated immediate hypersensitivity to a previously tolerated food following its avoidance for eosinophilic gastrointestinal diseases. J Allergy Clin Immunol Pract. 2018;6:649–50.

Kim EH, Burks AW. Food allergy immunotherapy: oral immunotherapy and epicutaneous immunotherapy. Allergy. 2020;75:1337–46.

Kim EH, Jones SM, Burks AW, Wood RA, et al. A 5-year summary of real-life dietary egg consumption after completion of a 4-year egg powder oral immunotherapy (eOIT) protocol. J Allergy Clin Immunol. 2020;145:1292–95.

Lieberman JA, Weiss C, Furlong TJ, Sicherer M, Sicherer SH. Bullying among pediatric patients with food allergy. Ann Allergy Asthma Immunol. 2010;105:282–86.

Maloney JM, Chapman MD, Sicherer SH. Peanut allergen exposure through saliva: assessment and interventions to reduce exposure. J Allergy Clin Immmunol. 2006; 118:719–24.

Nadeau KC, Schneider LC, Hoyte L, Borras I, Umetsu DT. Rapid oral desensitization in combination with omalizumab therapy in patients with cow's milk allergy. J Allergy Clin Immunol. 2011;127:1622–24.

Netting MJ, Middleton PF, Makrides M. Does maternal diet during pregnancy and lactation affect outcomes in offspring? a systematic review of food-based approaches. Nutrition. 2014;30:1225–41.

Nicolaides RE, Parrish CP, Bird JA. Food allergy immunotherapy with adjuvants. Immunol Allergy Clin North Am. 2020;40:149–73.

Nowak-Węgrzyn A, Chehade M, Groetch ME, Spergel JM, et al. International consensus guidelines for the diagnosis and management of food protein-induced enterocolitis syndrome: executive summary-workgroup report of the Adverse Reactions to Foods Committee, American Academy of Allergy, Asthma & Immunology. J Allergy Clin Immunol. 2017;139:1111–26.

Otani IM, Begin P, Kearney C, Dominguez TL, et al. Multiple-allergen oral immunotherapy improves quality of life in caregivers of food-allergic pediatric subjects. Allergy Asthma Clin Immunol. 2014;10:25. doi:10.1186/1710-1492-10-25.

Pepper AN, Assa'ad A, Blaiss M, Brown E, et al. Consensus report from the Food Allergy Research & Education (FARE) 2019 Oral Immunotherapy for Food Allergy Summit. J Allergy Clin Immunol. 2020;146: 244–49.

Perkin MR, Logan K, Tseng A, Raji B, et al. Randomized trial of introduction of allergenic foods in breast-fed infants. N Engl J Med. 2016;374: 1733–43.

Perkin MR, Togias A, Koplin J, Sicherer S. Food allergy prevention: more than peanut. J Allergy Clin Immunol Pract. 2020;8:1–13.

Pouessel G, Turner PJ, Worm M, Cardona V, et al. Food-induced fatal anaphylaxis: from epidemiological data to general prevention strategies. Clin Exp Allergy. 2018;48:1584–93.

Rank MA, Sharaf RN, Furuta GT, Aceves SS, et al. Technical review on the management of eosinophilic esophagitis: a report from the AGA Institute and the Joint Task Force on Allergy-Immunology Practice Parameters. Gastroenterology. 2020;158:1789–810.

Roberts G, Lack G. Relevance of inhalational exposure to food allergens. Curr Opin Allergy Clin Immunol. 2003;3:211–15.

Sakihara T, Otsuji K, Arakaki Y, Hamada K, Sugiura S, Ito K. Randomized trial of early infant formula introduction to prevent cow's milk allergy. J Allergy Clin Immunol. 2021;147:224–32.

Sampson HA, Aceves S, Bock SA, James J, et al. Food allergy: a practice parameter update—2014. J Allergy Clin Immunol. 2014;134:1016–25.

Savage J, Sicherer S, Wood R. The natural history of food allergy. J Allergy Clin Immunol Pract. 2016;4:196–203.

Schroer B, Groetch M, Mack DP, Venter C. Practical challenges and considerations for early introduction of potential food allergens for prevention of food allergy. J Allergy Clin Immunol Pract. 2021;9:44–56

Shemesh E, Annunziato RA, Ambrose MA, Ravid NL, et al. Child and parental reports of bullying in a consecutive sample of children with food allergy. Pediatrics. 2013;131:e10-17. doi:10.1542/peds.2012-1180.

Shemesh E, D'Urso C, Knight C, Rubes M, et al. Food-allergic adolescents at risk for anaphylaxis: a randomized controlled study of supervised injection to improve comfort with epinephrine self-injection. J Allergy Clin Immunol Pract. 2017;5:391–97.

Sicherer SH, Sampson HA. Food allergy: a review and update on epidemiology, pathogenesis, diagnosis, prevention, and management. J Allergy Clin Immunol. 2018;141:41–58.

Sicherer SH, Simons FE. Epinephrine for first-aid management of anaphylaxis. Pediatrics. 2017;139.

Sicherer SH, Furlong T, Maes HH, Desnick RJ, Sampson HA, Gelb BD. Genetics of peanut allergy: a twin study. J Allergy Clin Immunol. 2000;106:53–56.

Sicherer SH, Warren CM, Dant C, Gupta RS, Nadeau KC. Food allergy from infancy through adulthood. J Allergy Clin Immunol Pract. 2020;8:1854–64.

Simonte S, Ma S, Mofidi S, Sicherer SH. Relevance of casual contact with peanut butter in children with peanut allergy. J Allergy Clin Immunol. 2003;112:180–82.

Soller L, Mill C, Avinashi V, Teoh T, Chan ES. Development of anaphylactic cow's milk allergy following cow's milk elimination for eosinophilic esophagitis in a teenager. J Allergy Clin Immunol Pract. 2017; 5:1413–14.

Togias A, Cooper SF, Acebal M, Assa'ad A, et al. Addendum guidelines for the prevention of peanut allergy in the United States: report of the NIAID-sponsored expert panel. J Allergy Clin Immunol. 2017;139:29–44.

Umasunthar T, Leonardi-Bee J, Hodes M, Turner PJ, et al. Incidence of fatal food anaphylaxis in people with food allergy: a systematic review and meta-analysis. Clin Exp Allergy. 2013;43:1333–41.

Upton J, Nowak-Wegrzyn A. The impact of baked egg and baked milk diets on IgE- and non-IgE-mediated allergy. Clin Rev Allergy Immunol. 2018;55:118–38.

Urashima M, Mezawa H, Okuyama M, Urashima T, et al. Primary prevention of cow's milk sensitization and food allergy by avoiding supplementation with cow's milk formula at birth: a randomized clinical trial. JAMA Pediatr. 2019;173:1137–45.

Venter C, Sicherer SH, Greenhawt M. Management of peanut allergy. J Allergy Clin Immunol Pract. 2019;7:345–55.

Venter C, Greenhawt M, Meyer RW, Agostoni C, et al. EAACI position paper on diet diversity in pregnancy, infancy and childhood: novel concepts and implications for studies in allergy and asthma. Allergy. 2020;75:497–523.

Vickery BP, Vereda A, Casale TB, Beyer K, et al. AR101 oral immunotherapy for peanut allergy. N Engl J Med. 2018;379:1991–2001.

Wang J, Sicherer SH. Guidance on completing a written allergy and anaphylaxis emergency plan. Pediatrics. 2017;139. doi:10.1542/peds .2016-4005.

Waserman S, Cruickshank H, Hildebrand KJ, Mack D, et al. Prevention and management of allergic reactions to food in child care centers and schools: practice guidelines. J Allergy Clin Immunol. 2021 May;147: 1561–78.

Wasserman RL, Hague AR, Pence DM, Sugerman RW, et al. Real-world experience with peanut oral immunotherapy: lessons learned from 270 patients. J Allergy Clin Immunol Pract. 2019;7:418–26.

Weinberger T, Annunziato R, Riklin E, Shemesh E, Sicherer SH. A randomized controlled trial to reduce food allergy anxiety about casual exposure by holding the allergen: TOUCH study. J Allergy Clin Immunol Pract. 2019;7:2039–42.

Wood RA, Kim JS, Lindblad R, Nadeau K, et al. A randomized, double-blind, placebo-controlled study of omalizumab combined with oral immunotherapy for the treatment of cow's milk allergy. J Allergy Clin Immunol. 2016;137:1103–10.

Zeiger RS, Heller S, Mellon MH, Forsythe AB, O'Connor RD, Hamburger RN. Effect of combined maternal and infant food-allergen avoidance on development of atopy in early infancy: a randomized study. J Allergy Clin Immunol. 1989;84:72–89.

Index

blood disorders, 16, 48
blood pressure, low (hypotension), 9, 121, 145, 146, 148, 149
blood tests, 57, 59, 70–78, 84; for allergy resolution, 77, 226; anaphylaxis and, 67; for celiac disease, 8; for eosinophilic esophagitis, 153; false positive or false negative results, 71–72, 77; for FPIES, 145; in infants, 245–46; kIU/L or kU$_A$/L units, 71, 73, 74, 84, 95, 96; positive or negative results, 70, 72–73; skin tests vs., 67, 68, 69, 71, 73–74, 76
blood transfusions, 201–2
botulism, 46
bran, 28, 47
Brazil nuts, 29, 33, 79, 170
bread, 26, 34, 35, 36, 37, 47, 56, 133, 177, 280
breaded foods / breadcrumbs, 24, 28, 34
breastfeeding, 4, 199–200, 238–41, 242, 243, 250; allergy prevention and, 238–40; elimination diets during, 81, 143; food protein–induced proctocolitis and, 142–44; FPIES and, 149; infant colic and, 140
breath hydrogen test, 4, 5
breathing difficulties, 3, 9, 16, 102–3; anaphylaxis-related, 98, 99, 102–3, 108, 128, 129, 130
broccoli, 38, 147
brompheniramine, 58
bronchodilators, 119, 128, 129–30
Brussels sprouts, 38
BTK inhibitor (ibrutinib), 264
buckwheat, 28, 47
bullying, 182, 213–14
bumps/wheals, 66, 67, 70, 72
butter, 5, 26, 177

cabbage, 11, 38, 39
caffeine, 2, 6, 15
cake. See baked goods
calcium, 82, 217–18, 219, 220
calcium lactate, 27
camps, 192–93, 296–97
Canadian Society for Allergy and Clinical Immunology, 277
cancer, 8, 41
Candida, 285
candy, 22, 23, 24, 26, 27, 30–31, 46, 178
canned foods, 10–11, 24, 26, 35, 37, 41, 157
canola oil, 56, 216
capsaicin, 45
carbohydrates, 215, 216, 217, 219–20

carmine dye, 47, 48
carrageen, 42
carrots, 10, 37, 48, 219
casein, 25, 26, 27
cashews, 29–30, 32, 33, 39, 48, 51–52, 79, 170
cauliflower, 7, 11, 38, 147
caviar, 23, 43
celebrations and holidays, 178, 184–85
celery, 13, 16, 38, 105
celiac disease, 3, 6, 7–8, 28, 29, 150
cell-mediated food allergies, 2
cell phones, and ICE (In Case of Emergency) apps, 123
cellulose, 7
Centers for Disease Control and Prevention (CDC), 293
cereals, 26, 28, 30–31, 32, 34, 35, 247, 251, 252, 254
Caesarean section, 233–34
cetirizine (Zyrtec), 58, 117, 118
cheese, 4, 5, 15, 25, 26, 35, 56, 157, 161, 177, 184, 280
chef cards, 175, 176
chemicals: environmental exposure, 232–33; in foods, 2, 15, 16, 19, 38, 42, 47, 133, 156, 157. See also food additives and preservatives
chestnuts, 29, 39, 50, 170
chest tightness/pain, 99, 100, 141
chicken, 7, 23, 40, 82, 161, 167
chickpeas, 21, 36, 38
children, food allergies of, 2, 178; anaphylaxis, 128–30; anaphylaxis action plans, 122, 124–26; antihistamine dosage, 117; behavioral and developmental problems and, 14, 15; contact urticaria (hives), 13; diagnosis, 53; eosinophilic esophagitis, 152; epinephrine use in, 114, 115, 116; food allergy management responsibilities, 179, 182–83, 197–99; gut allergies, 12; oral food challenges, 88–89; prevalence, 18; restaurant meals, 177; self-management, 179, 181, 182–83; self-treatment, 182, 187, 189–90, 199; skin testing in, 66; symptoms, 9, 53; triggers, 2, 19
Chinese herbal medicine, 262
chinquapin, 170
chitin products, 44
chitosan, 44
chlorpheniramine, 58
chocolate(s), 15, 19, 22, 23, 26, 27, 30–31, 56, 157, 172
choking, 100, 121, 128, 129, 241, 247, 252

About the Author

Scott H. Sicherer, MD, is the Elliot and Roslyn Jaffe Professor of pediatric allergy and immunology at the Icahn School of Medicine at Mount Sinai and the Director of the Jaffe Food Allergy Institute. He is the Chief of the Division of Pediatric Allergy and Immunology and the Medical Director of the institution's Clinical Research Unit. Dr. Sicherer received his medical degree from the Johns Hopkins University School of Medicine and his pediatric training, including a chief residency, at Mount Sinai in New York City. He completed a fellowship in allergy and immunology at Johns Hopkins and then returned as a faculty member to Mount Sinai. He is board-certified in pediatrics and in allergy and immunology.

Dr. Sicherer's research interests, funded by the National Institutes of Health and Food Allergy Research & Education, include numerous aspects of food allergy, among them natural course, gastrointestinal manifestations, epidemiology, psychosocial and quality-of-life issues, diagnostics, prevention, modalities to educate physicians and patients, genetics, and treatments. He has published over 250 articles in scientific journals, authored numerous book chapters in major pediatric and allergy textbooks, edited 2 food allergy textbooks, and authored 6 food allergy books for the lay public. He has coauthored 20 reports from professional societies and government agencies providing guidance to allergists or pediatricians on approaching food allergy and anaphylaxis.

Dr. Sicherer served on the Committee on Food Allergies for the National Academies of Sciences. He is past chair of the Adverse Reactions to Foods Committee of the Academy of Allergy, Asthma, and Immunology (AAAAI); the Section on Allergy and Immunology of the American Academy of Pediatrics; and the board of directors of the American Board of Allergy and Immunology. He has served on the board of directors of the AAAAI and is deputy editor of the Journal of Allergy and Clinical Immunology: In Practice.

Dr. Sicherer has been consistently recognized as a "Top Doctor" by Castle-Connolly / New York Magazine, as among the top 1% of researchers in his field given the citation impact of his publications, and as among the top 1% of pediatric allergists according to U.S. News and World Report.

Printed in the USA
CPSIA information can be obtained
at www.ICGtesting.com
LVHW051948060324
773737LV00004B/161